Break Free From Migraines Naturally

Practical Steps to Reclaim Your Life and Prevent Migraines Effectively

Dr Sui H. Wong MD FRCP

EBH Press. EBHpress.com

Copyright © Dr Sui H. Wong, 2024

ISBN: 978-1-7385581-6-2 (Paperback) 978-1-917353-08-3 (E-book)

Audiobook : ASIN B0D84RG5PT

Table of Contents

Dedication

This book is dedicated to the migraine warriors I've had the privilege of guiding successfully, with lifestyle and holistic approaches to regain control of their lives and find freedom from migraines.

Introduction

Are you frequently experiencing headaches and you don't know why? Desperately looking for answers on how to prevent these from happening, fix your symptoms, and get some relief?

There is a specific reason why you're here today—most probably because you suffer from migraines and you want to get better. I decided to write this book for people who have migraines and want to find a complementary approach to regain control.

Studies show that about 90% of those who experience migraines look for alternative or complementary treatments (Kuruvilla et al., 2021). This book aims to share effective lifestyle and holistic approaches that can complement the care you are currently receiving. The information provided here is intended to empower you to be more involved in your migraine care.

At the same time, it encourages open communication and collaboration with your healthcare professionals as you embark on this complementary approach. The main goal is to give you a complete guide to help you find relief and improve your life by letting you understand migraines in a whole new way.

If this accurately describes you, it may encourage you to know that I wrote this book with you in mind. The lifestyle changes and information I'll share in these chapters will provide you with non-medical approaches to enhance your well-being. The power to improve your condition lies within you, and you can take control of your journey toward wellness.

Break Free From Migraines Naturally provides you with eight effective ways to better manage your migraines holistically. The book begins by providing an overview of headaches and migraines, and discusses the additional symptoms you may experience along with your migraines, as well as during the time before and after experiencing your headaches. We also look at the rationale for implementing foundational lifestyle factors such as best sleep practices, nutrition, emotional wellness, mindfulness, and hydration, and offer you valuable advice on how to do manage these factors.

We will explore evidence-informed practices from the holistic health sector that may not necessarily be considered mainstream in the medical world, but which have been reported to work and which I've found to be beneficial to my patients in my practice. This includes natural remedies and other alternative approaches that you may want to consider, especially if you can't use conventional medicine.

In *Break Free From Migraines Naturally*, you will find a comprehensive exploration of lifestyle-based approaches accompanied by practical tools for implementation, aimed at helping readers achieve a sustainable lifestyle that provides relief from headaches and migraines. Readers can experience improved mental clarity, mood, and overall wellbeing.

My objective is to empower you with the information you need to enjoy life, excel in your career, and foster meaningful connections with your loved ones—all without being hindered by frequent headaches and migraines.

By practising holistic self-care, you can find relief from frequent pain, allowing you to resume your normal life and maintain the positive lifestyle changes you've adopted. This will help you sustain and boost your brain health in the long term.

On this transformative exploration, we'll navigate the intricate landscape of holistic well-being, chapter by chapter. Here's a peek at what we're going to discuss:

- **The deal with migraines:** Uncover its origins and effective management strategies.

- **The pillars of sleep:** Delve into the profound impact of quality sleep and migraine prevention on overall wellness.

- **Exercise for migraine relief:** Discover exercise routine suggestions for alleviating migraines and embrace physical and mental vitality through somatic exercises, like yoga.

- **The gut-brain relationship:** Explore the complicated connection between gut health and brain function.

- **The relationship between female hormones and migraines:** Learn the common problems involving migraines during menstruation and menopause.

- **Metabolic factors and migraines:** Gain insights into metabolic contributors to headaches for a more informed health approach.

- **Nourishing your way to relief:** Understand how dietary choices can play a pivotal role in providing relief from headaches and migraines.

- **Utilizing practical tools and resources:** Equip yourself with valuable resources to enhance your well-being.

I am Dr. Sui H. Wong, and I'm thrilled to present this compelling work drawing from over two decades of medical expertise. As a seasoned medical doctor specializing in neurology and neuro-ophthalmology in the United Kingdom (UK), I have extensive experience in treating people with migraines. My deep commitment lies in empowering you, the reader, by providing high-quality health information and guiding you on a life-changing journey from illness to well-being.

As an integrative neurologist and physician, I incorporate evidence-based lifestyle medicine approaches to deliver person-centered care. With diverse qualifications that have informed my unique approach to effective migraine management, I am a proficient lifestyle and integrative medical doctor, a certified hypnotherapist, a yoga and mindfulness teacher, and a dedicated researcher. The prestigious recognition of Fellow of the Royal College of Physicians, UK, underscores my dedication to delivering excellence in patient care, with my clinical services awarded for their outstanding contributions.

In addition to my medical duties, I actively engage in neuroscience research, leading trials that aim to answer important questions and enhance patient-centered outcomes. My current focus involves pioneering research on lifestyle-based interventions for neurological conditions.

I'm honored to share this book, which draws from my successful use of personalized, lifestyle-based approaches to provide practical insights.

Today, I intend to share a holistic approach that will help you to manage your migraines without having to rely on more medication. This book offers alternatives according to what suits you best, thus fostering greater freedom of choice and freedom from pain.

Living with migraines can be an incredibly difficult and unpredictable journey. As someone who has worked closely with countless patients battling these debilitating headaches, I've witnessed firsthand the profound impact they can have on every aspect of life.

Migraines have a way of derailing even the best-laid plans without warning. The searing pain is only part of the battle—the non-headache symptoms like nausea, light and sound sensitivity, and mental fogginess can be just as challenging to navigate. As an invisible illness, it often leaves those battling its effects feeling deeply misunderstood by even their closest friends and family.

I've seen the strain migraines can put on relationships when the inability to be fully present with loved ones sets in. The cognitive challenges, from lapses in concentration to struggles with decision-making, can hinder productivity at work and school, leaving individuals feeling discouraged and overwhelmed. And the relentless fatigue and loss of energy that frequently accompany migraines can rob people of their spark and zest for life.

Believe me, I understand the frustration that comes with well-meaning advice like "Just cut out caffeine" or "Stop taking painkillers." If only it were that simple. Each person's experience with migraines is unique, and cookie-cutter solutions may not be effective.

That's why I've made it my mission to share an in-depth, personalized approach that has helped many of my patients regain control over their migraines. Through this book, I hope to equip you with the knowledge and practical strategies I've honed over years of clinical experience. We'll dive deep into the foundational aspects of migraine management, allowing you to tailor your approach to your specific needs and circumstances.

Now, I know medication is a large part of the puzzle for most people, but that's a conversation to have with your doctor. Here, we'll focus on the lifestyle modifications and holistic interventions that you can implement day-to-day. I'll point you toward reputable resources so you can research medication options if you wish, but my aim is to provide you with the tools to thrive without solely relying on pharmacological solutions.

Ultimately, I want you to feel acknowledged, listened to, and uplifted as you navigate this journey. I know how isolating and demoralizing migraines can be, but I also know that with the right guidance and unwavering commitment, you can mitigate their impact and reclaim your life. Together, we'll navigate this path toward renewed energy, productivity, and an overall improved quality of life—one step at a time.

So get ready for an evidence-informed exploration of holistic well-being. We're diving into headaches, sleep, exercise, the gut-brain connection, metabolic factors, hormones, and practical tools that will help you to enhance your health. Buckle up for a straightforward journey through the wellness essentials—no fluff, just facts. Let's get started on developing a more resilient, healthier you.

Chapter 1:
The Deal With Your Migraines

Meet our fictive migraine model, Sandy. She works as a graphic designer in the lively, fast-paced city of New York. Her days are filled with creativity, but there's a shadow hanging over her. There isn't a morning where the vibrant hues of her designs don't clash with the pounding pain in her head.

Sandy's is no ordinary headache. You guessed it—she faces migraines, each one bringing its own set of challenges. Some days, it's a full-blown migraine, and other times, it starts with warning signs like brain fog and problems concentrating. Explaining these experiences to co-workers becomes a daily struggle because, for Sandy, migraines are more than just headaches—they're a mix of confusing sensations.

Let's dive into the science of Sandy's migraines, exploring what's happening in her brain. It's a battleground where stress, family history, and everyday factors come together to trigger these throbbing headaches.

Speaking of family, Sandy's got a family tree full of migraines. She's dealing with headaches that have passed down through the generations, with her own lifestyle adding to it.

Her journey to brain resilience is about finding ways to fend off her daily migraines. We'll see how simple changes to her lifestyle and a focus on taking care of herself become important tools in her fight against these tough headaches.

In this chapter, we're going to take a deep dive into migraines. These are a common issue that affect many people, and we'll explore why they happen and how they impact us. Before we get into solutions, it's important to understand what headaches and migraines are, the different types of headaches and migraines, and their unique features. These conditions can be quite complex and are classified based on factors like how often they occur, how long they last, underlying causes, and additional symptoms they may cause.

Understanding Migraines

Across the globe, more than a billion people experience migraines every year (Amiri et al., 2022). Migraines, a disorder of the nervous system, are a specific kind of headache that often brings intense throbbing pain or a pulsing feeling, usually on just one side of your head. These typically last from four hours to three days and tend to happen about once to four times a month.

Sometimes, migraines come with other symptoms like nausea and visual disturbances, such as seeing flashes of light or having blind spots. Talking might also become a bit tricky during a migraine. Some people experience temporary neurological disturbance on one side of their body, which could include a tingling of the face or in an arm or leg. People can also get what is called a "silent migraine," which presents through the other symptoms mentioned above, without the headaches.

Almost anyone can experience a migraine if they encounter a sufficient number of triggers. Inadequate sleep, stress, dehydration, and alcohol consumption—these factors are the main culprits that can induce migraines in up to 90% of people (Mauskop, 2022).

While there is still much to learn, it is clear that migraines are a neurological condition involving a dysfunction in the brainstem's ability to regulate sensory information.

People who experience migraines may have difficulty controlling how their brain processes sensory inputs like sounds, lights, and smells. Studies have provided strong evidence supporting the idea that the brainstem is central to migraine attacks, as suggested by Goadsby et al. (2017).

During these attacks, the brainstem becomes overwhelmed and is unable to regulate sensory signals effectively, leading to an inability to filter out or ignore normal sensory stimuli. It's like someone cranked up the volume on all your senses to an unbearable level. Intense light, loud sounds, potent odors—things that wouldn't normally faze you suddenly become excruciating and triggering.

But why does this sensory overload happen in the first place? Researchers believe it has to do with the intricate network of neurons and pathways involved in processing sensory information (Goadsby et al., 2017). In migraine sufferers, there seems to be a disruption or hypersensitivity in this network, causing it to misfire and amplify even the mildest stimuli. Your genes could also play a role.

Imagine your brain is like a complex sound system, with various components working together to produce clear audio. In migraineurs, it's as if the equalizer is all out of whack, causing certain frequencies to become disproportionately amplified and distorted, leading to that overwhelming sensory experience.

Treating migraines could include taking medications, trying out self-help tips, and making lifestyle changes such as managing stress, exercising, and eating well. A holistic approach is the key to managing and overcoming this condition. And that's exactly what we will be discussing in this book.

The good news is that by understanding the root cause of migraines as a sensory processing disorder, researchers are paving the way for more targeted and effective treatments. Rather than just masking symptoms, future therapies could focus on rebalancing and "re-tuning" that sensory processing network in the brain.

What Is a Migraine?

I like this quotation from Professor Peter Goadsby (The Migraine Trust, n.d.). He's a world-leading migraine expert who has inspired me with his research and clinical care to patients. His quote sufficiently summarizes what a migraine is:

> Migraine is an inherited tendency to have headaches with sensory disturbance. It's an instability in the way the brain deals with incoming sensory information, and that instability can become

influenced by physiological changes like sleep, exercise and hunger.

Of course, this is just a simplified explanation of a very complex neurological process. But the key takeaway is that migraines aren't just bad headaches—they're a disorder of how the brain interprets and responds to the world around us. And by unraveling these mysteries of sensory processing, we're one step closer to finding better ways to manage and overcome this debilitating condition.

A migraine attack often brings with it numerous other symptoms. Nausea or vomiting, sensitivity to light or sound, tingling sensations in the skin, visual disturbances, slurred speech, and hunger can also manifest. During a migraine episode, almost everyone grapples with multiple symptoms. Abnormal brain biochemistry primarily causes migraines. Importantly, no one induces a migraine upon themselves; neither is it a psychological response to life issues or an unconscious wish to fall ill as an escape from daily challenges.

Migraines, on the other hand, often manifest due to genetic predisposition—one that can be inherited from either one or both parents. If both of your parents have it, your risk is even higher. A chronic condition, it defies cure and necessitates proactive management. Simply wishing away your migraine is an insufficient approach; instead, you must take deliberate steps to control it.

Diagnosing migraine accurately can take a while. Surprisingly, in the United States, only a quarter of people with migraines receive the correct diagnosis and appropriate treatment (Rizzoli, 2022). The rest are often told they have something like sinus problems, mental health conditions, dental issues, eye troubles, or just different types of headaches that will pass by themselves. Some don't even bother seeing a doctor about their symptoms. What's most interesting about migraines is that symptoms differ from one person to another.

Many factors can reduce your brain's resilience and trigger migraine attacks. This could be irregular sleep patterns, fluctuations in ovarian hormones, fasting, metabolic disturbances, poor sleep, prolonged stress, and lifestyle choices. Migraines are also way more common in women than in men, happening about three times as often.

Addressing these root causes and enhancing resilience through therapies may help reduce the frequency and intensity of migraines. You can't control or change your genes, but you can manage your environment. Later in this chapter, we'll talk more about the approaches we're going to cover in this book.

Now that you know a migraine is much more than a nasty headache, let's talk about the different symptoms, phases, and types of migraines people experience. You might identify your specific issue here, although you will still need to visit your doctor for an appropriate diagnosis.

Non-Headache Migraine Symptoms

Most often, other signs associated with migraines include:

- disturbances in vision, such as aura, flashes of light, or temporary vision loss.

- heightened sensitivity to stimuli such as light, sound, smells, touch, or motion.

- gastrointestinal issues like nausea, vomiting, and stomach discomfort.

- weakness, tingling, or feeling numb—often affecting one side of the body.

- feelings of dizziness, vertigo, or difficulty maintaining balance.

- cognitive challenges including confusion, concentration problems, difficulty with word recall, and mental fogginess.

- other manifestations such as food cravings, neck stiffness, profound fatigue, increased urination, and frequent yawning.

These symptoms may occur during or between migraine headache episodes, significantly impacting your daily functioning. Recognizing and addressing these non-headache manifestations is crucial for a comprehensive approach to managing your migraines.

Migraines Often Warn You in Advance

Migraines often send out sneak peeks before they strike in full force, like a movie trailer before the main event. Here are some common warning signs people experience:

- **Yawning:** If you're suddenly yawning a lot, it could be a heads-up that a migraine is on its way.

- **Stomach troubles:** Your tummy might start feeling off, with cramps or nausea creeping in.

- **Mood swings:** Your emotions might go on a rollercoaster ride, making you feel irritable, super happy, or maybe even panicky for no apparent reason.

- **Cravings:** Suddenly craving sweets or carbs? Your body might be trying to tell you that a migraine is about to hit.

- **A dry mouth and bathroom breaks:** You could start feeling extra thirsty and making more trips to the restroom.

- **Muscle tension:** Feeling stiff in your neck or shoulders could suggest a migraine is on its way.

Do you experience any of these symptoms before your migraine starts? Or do you experience any warning signs not listed here? Think of these as your body's early-warning system, giving you a heads-up to brace yourself for the migraine ahead.

There can also be other causes (not due to migraine) for these symptoms; the above is for education purposes and not meant to be a self-diagnosis list. This is something you will need to review together with your doctor.

Remember, every migraine experience is unique, and not everyone will go through all phases or exhibit the same symptoms. If you're dealing with migraines, talk to your doctor to tailor an effective management plan, including a holistic approach to build your brain's resilience.

Migraine Stages or Phases

Migraines don't just hit suddenly. For many people, they happen in distinct stages, with different symptoms at each stage. Not everyone goes through every stage, and symptoms can vary from person to person. However, understanding these typical stages can help you manage the migraine better.

It can be hard to determine when a migraine attack will happen. Nevertheless, the distinct stages of each attack often follow a pattern that you will start recognizing if you are mindful. The distinct symptoms of these stages differentiate a migraine from a headache.

In adults, a migraine attack can be categorized into four to five sequential stages (Healthdirect, n.d.; *Stages of a migraine attack*, n.d.):

- **Prodromal (pre-monitory):** This can start up to one to two days before the migraine headache kicks in, and you may experience some of the warning signs we discussed in the previous section. You might feel tired, irritable, have a stiff neck, or feel anxious. Yawning and mood swings are common. Some people even get food cravings, like chocolate.

- **Aura:** Not everyone gets this, but for those who do, it's usually visual changes like flashing lights or zigzags. Sometimes, people might feel dizzy or have trouble speaking. Typically, this occurs right before the headache begins.

- **Headache or pain (main attack):** This is when the migraine headache hits. It persists for a duration ranging from 4 to 72 hours and manifests as pulsating pain. It's not just pain; it can also make you feel sick and sensitive to light and sound.

- **Resolution:** Most occurrences gradually go away, while a few stop abruptly. A short nap can help with this.

- **Postdrome:** Commonly known as a migraine hangover, this stage succeeds the headache and can extend for several hours and up to 48. Symptoms might entail exhaustion, challenges with focus, and heightened sensitivity to touch, light, and sound. After the headache goes away, you might still feel kind of foggy and tired for up to five days, and sometimes people feel like they're getting another migraine before they fully recover.

Some people might not experience certain phases like aura, while others might have different symptoms or recovery times. For some people, the headache is very mild, more like a "heaviness" in their head, but the other symptoms are more prominent and troublesome. For some, the symptoms in each stage may even overlap.

Recognizing the various phases of a migraine attack can be beneficial as they may vary in duration and intensity, but identifying specific symptoms at specific times during an attack can provide valuable information to the doctor for diagnosis. Taking action promptly upon noticing the pain can potentially halt or reduce the duration of the attack. In children, migraine attacks are typically briefer than in adults, making it easier to distinguish between the headache stages.

Types of Migraines

Even though migraine impacts nearly 40 million people in the United States (Migraine Research Foundation, n.d.), the symptoms look different from one person to another.

- **Migraine without aura:** The most common type, characterized by intense, pulsating head pain typically on one side, lasting for hours to days. People might also experience other symptoms like tiredness, vomiting, vision changes such as seeing flashing lights or wavy lines, becoming more irritable, and difficulty handling light or sound that is too bright or loud, respectively.

- **Migraine with aura:** Preceded by sensory disturbances known as aura, such as flashing lights, visual changes, or a feeling indicating an impending migraine attack.

- **Chronic migraine:** Occurs when migraines happen on 15 or more days per month for at least three months, indicating a chronic condition.

- **Abdominal migraine:** Mainly present in children struggling with symptoms such as nausea, vomiting, and abdominal pain.

- **Hemiplegic migraine:** A rare but extreme form of migraine that includes temporary paralysis or weakness on one side of the body during the aura phase.

- **Retinal migraine:** Results in temporary vision loss or visual disturbances affecting one eye. Migraines with visual auras are often misdiagnosed as retinal migraines, where the visual disturbance affects both eyes when each eye is tested individually by covering one eye at a time. In other words, in retinal migraine, the migraine affects the retina, whereas in visual aura the migraine affects the visual cortex of the brain.

- **Vestibular migraine:** Experiencing symptoms of loss of balance and dizziness.

- **Menstrual migraine:** Linked to hormonal changes during the menstrual cycle. These migraines are a direct result of a decline in estrogen levels (Barth et al., 2015).

- **Acephalgic (silent) migraine:** Characterized by aura symptoms without the usual headache pain.

What Can Trigger Your Migraine?

Migraines start with an imbalance of sensory control in your midbrain. Certain things can trigger migraines, like lights, sounds, smells, or movement. People with migraines tend to be more sensitive to these things even when they're not having an attack.

Below are some examples of the things that can trigger migraines:

- **Physical activity:** Pushing yourself too hard with exercise or other physical activities can bring on a migraine.

- **Food additives:** Additives like nitrates or MSG found in cured meats and vegetables or processed foods might trigger migraines.

- **Addictive substances:** Consuming caffeine or tobacco products can sometimes trigger migraines.

- **Alternative remedies:** While some herbal supplements or practices may help with migraines, others could trigger them in some individuals.

- **Sensory difficulties:** Extreme noise, intense smells, or bright lights can overwhelm your senses and lead to a migraine.

Overall, migraines are pretty complex, and there's still a lot we don't fully understand about them. However, knowing the different stages and being aware of your migraine triggers can help you manage them better.

Managing Migraines: A Holistic Approach

Migraines can feel like an uphill battle, but this book aims to equip you with a comprehensive strategy to manage them.

Dealing with migraines can be challenging, but there are ways to manage them beyond relying solely on medication. Migraines signal when your body is out of balance and suggest necessary actions to restore your well-being.

In my Migraine-free BRA(i)NS® mentorship program, I take a systematic approach to overcoming migraines. This includes getting good sleep, eating healthy, managing your blood sugar, taking care of your gut (which greatly impacts your brain), ensuring you get the right nutrients, and staying active.

But that's not all—we also dive into techniques that help bring your ANS, which controls things like your heart rate and breathing, into balance. This is super important because when this system gets out of balance, it can trigger migraines. So, we'll look at vagus nerve activation through practices like yoga, mindfulness meditation, and breathwork exercises that teach you to keep calm and carry on, even when things get stressful.

By combining these approaches—building up your brain's strength and finding that inner balance—you'll be better equipped to prevent migraines from taking over your life. Remember, it's all about giving your body and mind the tools they need to work together harmoniously, rather than letting your migraines call the shots.

While there is no cure for migraine at the moment, there are reliable strategies available to help you manage pain and reduce the frequency of your attacks. These could include using over-the-counter pain relievers like ibuprofen or aspirin, prescription medications, surgery, lifestyle adjustments, and alternative therapies such as cognitive-behavioral therapy.

Imagine you have a pot of water on the stove starting to boil. The boiling pot represents migraines that someone is prone to because of their genes. It's like the heat is already turned on, and the water is bubbling.

Now, there are two main ways to deal with this boiling pot situation, just like there are two approaches to managing migraines.

- **Adding cool water:** This is like taking medication for migraine relief. When you add cool water to the boiling pot, it temporarily lowers the temperature and calms down the boiling. Similarly, medications like ibuprofen, aspirin, or prescription drugs can provide temporary relief from a migraine attack by reducing the pain and symptoms.

- **Turning down the heat**: This is like making lifestyle changes and trying natural remedies. Instead of just adding cool water, you can turn down the heat source under the pot to prevent it from boiling over in the first place. In the same way, making changes to your diet, reducing stress, practising relaxation techniques like mindfulness, and identifying triggers can help reduce the frequency and severity of migraine attacks. It addresses the root cause instead of just providing temporary relief.

The key is that while medications (like the analogy of adding cool water) can help during a migraine attack, lifestyle changes and natural remedies (like the analogy of turning down the heat) can help prevent the attacks from happening as often or from getting as severe. It's about managing the underlying condition, not just treating the symptoms.

The aim of this book isn't to coach you on medicine use or provide you with any medical advice, which is a matter you are best to discuss with your treating doctor. We will instead hone in on a holistic approach that will include important tips to strengthen your brain's resilience.

Get ready to learn life-changing strategies that will leave you feeling empowered and in control, instead of being at the mercy of your dreaded migraine attacks.

Building a Foundation for Brain Resilience

A key focus will be nurturing your brain's resilience through critical lifestyle factors.

- **Sleep:** We'll look at the vital role of quality sleep and develop habits to improve your rest.

- **Physical activity:** You'll learn how to leverage the power of movement to reduce migraine frequency and boost overall well-being.

- **Nutrition:** We'll find out how a migraine-friendly diet and specific nutrients can nourish and protect your brain.

- **Metabolic Health:** You'll learn the effect of blood sugar fluctuations and metabolic health on your migraine frequency, and how to manage this.

- **Supplements:** We'll demystify vitamins, minerals, and supplements that may benefit migraine management.

- **Gut-brain health:** You'll discover the fascinating connection between your gut and brain health, and how to nurture this vital link.

Restoring Autonomic Balance

From my experience, balancing the ANS is an important part of preventing migraines. The ANS is the part of the nervous system that controls the "automatic" functions of your body, for example, heartbeat, blood pressure, and even sweating. There are two parts to this—the "fight/flight" (also called sympathetic) and "rest/relax" (also called the parasympathetic) parts of the ANS, or the autonomic nervous system. When this system is out of balance, like when someone is excessively stressed, they may be stuck in "fight/flight," which can make it more likely for them to get migraines.

Your ANS acts like your body's control tower, regulating heart rate and digestion functions. When imbalanced, migraines become more likely. We'll explore techniques to restore this equilibrium.

- **Mindfulness:** Learn to utilize present-moment awareness to calm the mind and ease physical tension.

- **Breathwork, yoga, and mind-body practices:** Rediscover ancient wisdom to unify your mind, body, and breathing.

With resilience and autonomic balance as core focuses, we'll navigate the following to help us achieve the results we long for:

- **Hormones:** Understand how hormonal fluctuations interplay with migraine patterns and promote balance.

- **Complementary therapies:** Explore holistic practices like acupuncture and massage for additional support.

- **Trigger identification:** Develop strategies to recognize and avoid your unique migraine triggers.

By fortifying your lifestyle foundations with these holistic practices, you'll raise your migraine threshold and reclaim your freedom to live fully, unencumbered by debilitating attacks.

Concerns About Your Brain Health

Because migraine is a neurological condition, people often ask me if they should be concerned about their brain health. While brain imaging of people with migraines may sometimes reveal alterations or lesions, these changes are often of no significant concern. They can occasionally resemble minor blood flow changes but are typically not associated with cognitive impairment or an increased risk of stroke. However, if you have concerns about any brain imaging findings related to your migraines, discussing them with a neurologist for a proper evaluation and explanation is recommended.

Is a Brain Scan Necessary if You Have Frequent Migraines?

Whether you believe you need a brain scan or your general practitioner (GP) has recommended that you undergo one, this remains something that you are best to discuss with your doctor. Typically, if you have been diagnosed with migraines, have undergone a normal physical examination, and there are no other alarming symptoms, such as a sudden severe headache (commonly known as a thunderclap headache) or a new headache if you are over 50, a brain scan is usually unnecessary.

A Brief Note About Medication Overuse Headache

Beware of the risk of developing medication overuse headache if you are using painkillers or triptans for migraines, for more than 15 days a month over a period of longer than 3 months. In my clinical practice, I often see the inadvertent development of this type of headache, on top of the existing migraine headaches, due to the amount of painkillers used. Please discuss this with your doctor if this is relevant to you.

Key Takeaways

Now, let's reinforce your knowledge and recap what we've talked about in Chapter 1:

- Migraines are a distinct neurological condition, not just severe headaches. They involve a complex set of symptoms beyond head pain alone.

- Migraines often occur in phases—prodrome, aura, attack, postdrome—with a variety of potential symptoms like sensory disturbances, nausea, fatigue, and cognitive difficulties.

- Many potential triggers can set off a migraine attack, including hormonal changes, stress, lack of sleep, certain foods, and sensory stimuli.

- Recognizing the early warning signs and promptly managing triggers can help reduce the severity and duration of migraine attacks.

- While migraines are not life-threatening, they can significantly impact daily life, warranting proper medical evaluation and a personalized treatment plan.

- A holistic approach addressing lifestyle factors like sleep, nutrition, exercise, and stress management complements medical treatment for better migraine control.

- Comprehending the complexity of migraines is vital for correct diagnosis, personalized management, and improved well-being for those affected.

The uncertainty of when your next migraine might strike can lead to constant fear and disrupt your work, family, and social responsibilities. It's important to understand the challenging concept of different headaches and migraines for pain control, correct management, and a higher quality of life.

*****

The upcoming chapter will delve into the element of sleep and its significant effects on your wellness.

Chapter 2:
The Pillars of Sleep

Sleep is one of the foundational aspects of brain health. Improving the quality and/or duration of your sleep is a great way to start building brain resilience and prevent migraines.

In this chapter, we explore the fundamentals that form the pillars of sleep. Sleep isn't about taking a break; it's a necessary task that greatly influences our health and overall well-being. We'll explore why sleep is so important, its different stages, and the factors that can either enhance or disrupt our sleep quality. Come along as we uncover the vital secrets to help you create a healthy sleep environment.

Understanding the Stages of Sleep

You may think bedtime is as easy as going to sleep and waking up the next morning, but there's more! Sleep is an intricate process, having different stages, each with its responsibility in helping your body heal. There are primarily two categories of sleep stages: rapid eye movement (REM), and non-rapid eye movement (NREM) sleep (Pacheco & Singh, 2023). These stages take turns in cycles that last about an hour and a half each. Let's discuss these stages so you can get a better picture of how it works.

Different Sleep Stages

Your sleep cycle is made up of four stages, interchanging from NREM to REM sleep throughout the night. Let's explore them (Harvard Health Publishing, n.d.):

- **Stage 1—Light NREM sleep:** This stage happens when we shift from being awake to entering sleep mode and lasts up to five minutes. Your breathing and heart rate become somewhat slower.

- **Stage 2—Deeper NREM sleep:** Now, your body temperature decreases and your heart rate drops even more. Your brain waves increase in frequency, occasionally showing rapid bursts. Your muscles relax more, too. This stage typically constitutes over half of adult sleep time and extends with each sleep cycle.

- **Stage 3—Deepest NREM sleep:** Waking up from this stage of sleep is the most difficult to do. During this stage, your body's functions are at their slowest pace. This stage typically lasts no more than 40 minutes at most, after which your body moves to the last phase of sleep.

- **Stage 4—REM sleep:** In this phase, your brain becomes more active as your brain waves increase in frequency, occasionally showing bursts of waves. This stage typically accounts for over half of an adult's sleep time and extends in duration with each sleep cycle.

During the last two stages of sleep, your body repairs tissues, strengthens bones and muscles and boosts the immune system. These phases help your body recover.

Once the NREM and the REM stages are complete, the cycle starts over. This happens around every 80 to 100 minutes. In most cases, you have about four to six sleep cycles each night and you may wake up briefly in the middle of these cycles (NIH, 2022).

The Importance of Sleeping

Improving sleep is one of the key components that has helped many of my patients, enhancing their brain resilience and reducing the likelihood of triggers bringing on migraines.

Before we concentrate on sleep and migraines, let's first find out why sleep is so important in your daily life. Sleep is a precious gem when it comes to staying healthy and feeling good. It's one of the main pillars of health, along with eating well and staying active, to keep your body's house standing. These pillars are all connected and important for keeping us healthy.

Sleep is crucial for our emotional health. The body's internal clock, which controls when we sleep and wake up, is linked to many important functions like our body temperature, hormones, and immune system. If our sleep schedule is disrupted, it can raise the risk of heart problems, metabolic disorders, and cancer.

Keeping our brain and mental health in check requires that we combine holistic approaches including sleep, physical activity, mindful thinking, and managing our emotions. When we don't sleep like we should, all these other factors are affected in some way.

To support brain health and prevent memory loss as we get older, good sleep is one of the key things we can do to help keep our brains sharp and lower our chances of getting diseases like Alzheimer's.

In short, sleep is a major player in our health. Making sure we get enough quality sleep can make a big difference in how we feel and how healthy we stay.

The Role of Sleep in Overall Health and Well-Being

Sleep is not merely a passive state; it has an important job to do, as we established in the previous section. Here are some key reasons why quality sleep matters (Harvard Health Publishing, n.d.):

- **Metabolic health:** Poor sleep is linked to weight gain, insulin resistance, and an increased risk of diabetes and obesity.

- **Physical restoration:** During sleep, our body engages in tissue repair, growth, and immune system maintenance. Lack of sleep can impair these processes, leading to increased vulnerability to illnesses.

- **Cardiovascular well-being:** Insufficient sleep raises your risk of heart disease, hypertension, and stroke.

- **Cognitive function:** Sleep is essential for memory consolidation, learning, and problem-solving. It enhances creativity, focus, and decision-making abilities.

- **Emotional well-being:** Adequate sleep contributes to stable mood, emotional resilience, and stress management. Chronic sleep deprivation can exacerbate anxiety and depression.

- **Controlling inflammation:** Sleep helps regulate inflammation in the body. Chronic inflammation is associated with various health conditions.

Sleeping helps to keep your heart strong, boost your memory, improve your executive functioning, manage your weight, support your immune system, and promote emotional well-being. These benefits highlight the significance of making quality sleep a priority for your well-being (Stibich, 2023).

Sleep and Migraines

By prioritizing sleep hygiene, establishing a consistent sleep routine, and ensuring adequate sleep duration, you can support your overall health, and potentially reduce the frequency and severity of migraine attacks. Adequate sleep should be considered an essential component of a comprehensive migraine management plan. Here's why.

Circadian Rhythm and Regularity

Your body's circadian rhythm, or internal clock, regulates many physiological processes, including sleep-wake cycles. Disruptions in the circadian rhythm can trigger migraines or exacerbate their symptoms.

Maintaining a regular sleep schedule is crucial for migraine management, as it helps synchronize the body's internal clock and improves your brain's resilience against other migraine triggers.

The Relationship Between Circadian Rhythm and Sleep

Our sleep-wake cycles and overall alertness levels are regulated by a finely tuned system (homeostasis). When this delicate balance is thrown off, the system tries to make amends and restore equilibrium.

A migraine attack might represent an extreme and abnormal overcompensation mechanism employed by your body to correct this imbalance. For instance, if you're sleep-deprived, a migraine attack may force you to lie down in a dark, quiet environment, compelling you to rest. This may be your body's need to temporarily "power down and reset" because of sensory overload.

Understanding the Circadian Rhythm and Melatonin: To Help You Sleep Better

We spoke about the circadian rhythm as your body's internal clock that regulates your sleep-wake cycle. A study that systematically reviewed past studies on the timing of migraines has shown that mornings tend to be the most frequent peak onset (Poulsen et al., 2021), a pattern that suggests there might be a timing mechanism linked to sleep or our body's circadian rhythm.

Lack of sleep is a well-known migraine trigger, but interestingly enough, even too much sleep, like sleeping in on weekends, can also provoke an attack. For some people, disruptions in their sleep-wake cycle due to working irregular hours or jet lag from traveling can increase the likelihood of experiencing a migraine, implying that both sleep and the circadian timing system play a role (Walker et al., 2020).

Right before a migraine attack, excessive sleepiness is a common symptom (The Migraine Trust, n.d.–a). Conversely, after an attack, some people may experience a similar feeling of extreme drowsiness.

Interestingly, getting a good night's sleep can often alleviate or even stop a migraine attack.

Your circadian rhythm is influenced by environmental cues, such as light and darkness, and is also controlled by the release of hormones like melatonin.

Melatonin is a hormone made by the pineal gland in the brain. Its release is mainly affected by the intensity of light exposure. When it gets dark, melatonin levels naturally increase, signaling to the body that it's time to sleep. Conversely, when exposed to bright light, and specifically blue light from electronics, melatonin production is suppressed, promoting wakefulness.

The relationship between melatonin and the circadian rhythm is crucial for maintaining a healthy sleep-wake cycle. Disruptions in this rhythm, caused by irregular sleep patterns, exposure to blue light at night, or other factors, can affect melatonin release and contribute to sleep disturbances, which are known migraine triggers for many people.

If you struggle to fall asleep, taking melatonin as a supplement can help you. It's essential to consult with your doctor before starting any supplementation, especially if you have pre-existing medical conditions or if you are taking other medications. Your doctor can guide the appropriate dosage and timing of melatonin supplements to ensure safe and effective use.

Toxin Clearance and Brain Health

During deep sleep, the brain undergoes a process called glymphatic clearance, where metabolic waste and toxins are flushed out. Inadequate sleep can impair this much-needed cleansing process, leading to the accumulation of potentially harmful substances.

Both cluster headaches and migraines appear to involve some dysregulation or abnormalities in REM sleep, either as a trigger or consequence of the headache disorders. Migraine sufferers experience more disruptions during the REM stage and abnormal cycling patterns compared to healthy individuals. Collectively, these findings suggest potential dysfunction in the brainstem networks responsible for regulating the transitions between sleep stages (Vgontzas & Pavlović, 2018).

Blood Sugar Regulation

Sleep plays an important part in controlling your blood sugar levels and insulin sensitivity. Frequent changes in blood sugar can trigger migraines or worsen existing symptoms. Adequate sleep helps maintain stable blood sugar levels, which is an essential aspect of migraine prevention and management strategies.

Emotional Regulation and Stress Resilience

Sleep deprivation can affect emotional regulation, heighten stress levels, and reduce resistance to triggers. Chronic stress and emotional distress are known migraine triggers for many individuals. Quality sleep promotes emotional well-being, enhances stress coping mechanisms, and may help prevent migraine attacks triggered by psychological factors.

Sleep-Related Conditions

Certain sleep disorders and conditions can affect sleep quality—you may benefit from discussing with your healthcare professional if this is a concern for you. Some common ones are listed below.

Sleep Apnea

Characterized by interrupted delivery of oxygen to the lungs, sleep apnea may stem from a brain disorder (central sleep apnea) or the collapse of your airways during rest—an event often related to being overweight. Symptoms might manifest as snoring and gasping for air in nocturnal moments; consequently, this could compromise quality slumber and induce daytime fatigue. Through an overnight stay in a sleep laboratory or the utilization of a take-home device, diagnosis can be confirmed. Treatment options encompass weight loss, oral appliance usage, surgery to eradicate excess tissue that obstructs airflow, and finally, either continuous positive airway pressure (CPAP) machine application or Inspire implantable device use in certain situations.

Restless Leg Syndrome (RLS)

Another common condition (often undiagnosed) can that disrupt sleep and trigger migraines manifests as constant foot shaking or excessive leg movements during sleep. Iron and vitamin B12 deficiencies can exacerbate RLS. A sleep study and the elimination of these deficiencies form part of the diagnosis process. If you think you may have RLS, please make an appointment with your medical doctor for an assessment.

Insomnia

Insomnia—difficulty falling asleep or staying asleep—is a common issue for many migraine sufferers. This can be due to various factors, including pain, anxiety, stress, and depression. However, several non-drug therapies can help improve sleep quality without resorting to medication. Consider visiting a sleep specialist for a review if you are severely affected by insomnia.

Understanding Blue Light: How Screens Affect Your Sleep and Headaches

Blue light is a type of light that comes from screens on devices like phones, tablets, and computers. When you look at these screens, especially at night, it can mess up your body's natural sleep clock and make it hard to sleep well.

How Blue Light Disrupts Your Sleep

Blue light can stop your body from making melatonin. It can also make your sleep less restful by reducing the deep sleep your brain needs to feel refreshed.

Blue Light and Migraines

Looking at screens too much, especially before bed, might make you more likely to get headaches or migraines. This could be because blue light messes with your body's sleep cycle and how your brain reacts to light.

Ways to Prevent Blue Light Overexposure

- Try to use screens less, especially before bed.

- Use apps or settings on your devices that reduce blue light.

- Make a bedtime routine that doesn't involve screens, like reading a book or listening to music.

By being mindful of how much blue light you're exposed to, you can improve your sleep and lower your chances of getting headaches or migraines.

How to Optimize Your Sleep

Understanding the connection between sleep and migraines is necessary for effective management and holistic treatment. Almost all of us have struggled with sleep at some point. Unfortunately, when it comes to migraines, this bedtime story goes a little deeper. People who experience migraines are significantly more prone to encountering sleep-related issues. For instance, insomnia affects half or three-quarters of those persons with persistent pain and headache disorders such as migraines. Moreover, the quality of sleep is closely associated with specific types of headaches, like hypnic and cluster headaches (American Migraine Foundation, 2022).

What's behind all of this? Circadian rhythm drives our 24-hour sleep-and-wake cycle (Reddy et al., 2023). Some migraine patients experience changes in biomarkers that influence their sleep cycle, including cortisol during the day and melatonin at night. This could be a reason why they're more susceptible to disruptions in their sleep patterns.

The positive news is that you can enhance your sleep-wake cycle by developing healthy bedtime routines, such as going to bed consistently at set times, getting sunlight exposure in the morning, and refraining from using screens (like televisions, tablets, laptops, and mobile phones) before sleeping.

Let's talk about how you can improve your sleep environment and nightly routine for a better night's sleep.

Enhancing Your Sleep Environment and Routine

Improving your sleep quality starts with creating the right environment and sticking to a routine. Establishing healthy sleep habits, known as sleep hygiene, is crucial for improving the quality of your sleep. These practices involve setting up a consistent bedtime and wake-up time every day. This helps regulate your body's internal clock, making it easier for you to fall asleep and wake up naturally. Here are some tips to help you get a better night's rest:

Create a Sleep-Friendly Environment

Your bedroom should be quiet, dark, and kept at a comfortable temperature. This can tell your body that it's time to sleep. Invest in a comfortable mattress and pillows—a proper mattress can make a big difference in how well you sleep.

Avoiding screens and stimulating activities before bedtime can also help prepare your body for sleep.

When migraineurs incorporate these non–drug therapies into their routine, they can improve their sleep quality and overall well–being without over-reliance on medication.

Keep to a Regular Sleep Schedule

Consistency is key. Many migraineurs benefit from maintaining a consistent sleep schedule, even on weekends. Anticipating extra sleep on weekends may lead to disappointment for some; they might trigger a migraine by sleeping in.

If you find yourself needing more rest, consider taking a short nap in the afternoon, but keep it under an hour. Sleeping in and experiencing sudden relief from the week's constant stress are two common causes of weekend migraine attacks. Try to go to bed and wake up at the same time every day. This can help control your body's clock.

Limit Screen Time Before Bed

We've discussed how the blue light from screens can interrupt your body's production of melatonin. Try to limit your screen time prior to bedtime, or use blue light filters on your devices. Ideally, avoiding the use of electronic gadgets in your bedroom at all is the best approach.

Improving Your Lifestyle Habits

While medication can provide some form of relief from migraine, making lifestyle changes is an equally important part of managing this condition. Simple changes to your daily habits and routines can have a positive effect on reducing migraine frequency and severity. When you manage factors like sleep, stress, diet, and exercise, you'll be better equipped to keep migraines at bay and improve your overall well-being. Let's explore some effective lifestyle strategies for improved sleep.

Cognitive-Behavioral Therapies (CBT)

CBT is a type of therapy that focuses on changing negative thought patterns and behaviors that may contribute to insomnia. It can help migraine sufferers identify and address the underlying causes of their sleep difficulties, leading to improved sleep quality over time.

Natural Remedies

Certain natural remedies have been shown to promote better sleep in migraine sufferers. Magnesium, for example, is a mineral that assists with muscle relaxation and may improve sleep quality. Herbal teas like chamomile or valerian may help promote relaxation and improve sleep quality. Melatonin, as mentioned earlier, is a hormone that helps regulate sleep-wake cycles and can be useful for improving sleep in migraine sufferers. You may even consider taking pistachios, as a natural food source of melatonin. However, talk to a healthcare provider before starting any supplement regimen.

Practice Relaxation Techniques

Deep breathing, meditation, or progressive muscle relaxation can help reduce stress and promote better sleep. Discover a wealth of mindfulness resources in my books, complete with audioguides for enhanced experience. Refer to the Appendix at the end of this book for further details.

Try incorporating these techniques into your bedtime routine. Visualization and guided imagery techniques involve focusing on calming and positive images to help relax the mind and body. These techniques can be particularly helpful for migraine sufferers who experience anxiety or stress that may contribute to insomnia. We will discuss these relaxation techniques in more detail in Chapter 5 when we talk about stress management.

Focus on Nutrition for Sleep

Foods rich in tryptophan, like turkey, dairy, and nuts, can promote restful sleep. Tryptophan is an amino acid that helps your body produce serotonin, a neurotransmitter that regulates sleep. Magnesium-rich foods, such as leafy greens and nuts, can also help you relax and better your sleep quality.

It is crucial to refrain from consuming caffeine, large meals, and alcohol before going to bed. These substances can disrupt your sleep patterns and make it harder to fall asleep.

Get Regular Exercise

Engaging in regular physical activity during the day can help regulate your body's sleep-wake cycle, leading to improved overall sleep quality at night (CDC, 2022).

By incorporating these sleep hygiene practices into your daily routine, you can improve the quality of your sleep and wake up feeling refreshed and rejuvenated each day. These practices not only improve your sleep quality but also contribute to your overall well-being.

Key Takeaways

- **Why sleep matters:** Sleep is super important for your health. It helps your body heal, keeps your heart strong, boosts your memory, manages your weight, supports your immune system, and keeps your mood stable.

- **Sleep and migraines:** Keeping a regular sleep schedule and dealing with sleep problems like sleep apnea and restless leg syndrome can help reduce the frequency of your migraines. If you have trouble sleeping, there are ways to improve your sleep without medication.

- **Circadian rhythm:** Disrupted circadian rhythms from irregular sleep patterns, shift work, or jet lag can trigger migraines. Maintaining a consistent sleep-wake schedule helps align the body's internal clock.

- **Melatonin, magnesium, and other natural remedies:** Melatonin is a hormone that helps you know when to sleep and wake up. Taking melatonin, magnesium, and other natural remedies can help you sleep better and might even reduce how often you experience migraines.

- **Blue light and sleep:** Blue light from screens can disrupt your sleep and make you more likely to get headaches or migraines. Try to use screens less before bed to improve your sleep.

- **Tips for better sleep:** Create a peaceful sleep environment, stick to a regular sleep schedule, limit screen time before bed, practice relaxation techniques, and eat foods that help you sleep better. These habits can improve your sleep and reduce how often you get migraines.

In closing, prioritizing good sleep habits is crucial, as it can help prevent migraines , and enhance your overall well-being.

*****

Next, we'll zoom in on how physical activity, including exercises such as yoga, can play a role in alleviating your migraines.

Chapter 3:
Exercise for Migraine Relief

Living with migraines can be a rollercoaster. Despite the ups and downs, many people are determined not to let migraines take over their lives or keep them from staying healthy. Understanding and managing migraines is key, and adding exercise to your routine can be a great way to support your brain health and manage migraines.

Exercise is hailed as a key component of a healthy lifestyle, offering numerous benefits for both your body and mind. But for those who experience migraines, the relationship with exercise can be quite intricate. While regular physical activity has been shown to lessen the frequency and intensity of migraines for some, others find that certain types of exercise can trigger or worsen their symptoms.

In this chapter, we'll delve into the role of exercise in managing migraines, exploring the potential advantages, common triggers, and best approaches for integrating exercise into your migraine care routine. By learning how exercise can impact migraines, you can make informed choices for your physical routine to improve your overall well-being.

Does Exercise Help With Migraines?

Adding exercise to your routine could be a beneficial approach to managing symptoms and reducing the frequency of attacks. While research results may vary, there is supporting evidence for incorporating mild to moderate exercise as part of a comprehensive plan to treat migraines.

The Benefits of Aerobic Exercise for Migraines

Getting active is a part of staying healthy, and for people dealing with migraines, it can really make a difference. The latest Physical Activity

Guidelines for Americans from the U.S. Department of Health and Human Services (HHS, 2018) advise that regular aerobic exercise is beneficial for everyone, including those with migraines.

Exercise is an alternative for the preventative treatment of migraine if you are not benefiting from medication or for some reason cannot take or prefer not to take medication on a daily basis. (Varkey et al., 2011). Combining exercise with the other lifestyle strategies covered in this book is a winning recipe to conquer your migraines.

The emphasis on exercise stems from its impact on pain-processing mechanisms. When exercising, the body releases endorphins, which function as natural pain relievers.

Engaging in regular aerobic exercise could result in a decrease in the frequency of migraine episodes, along with reduced levels of pain (Lemmens et al., 2019). Activities like cycling and walking may be more suitable for people with migraines compared to high-intensity exercises involving muscle building (Amin et al., 2018).

Can Exercise Trigger Migraine Attacks?

It's possible. According to a study (Koppen & Van Veldhoven, 2013), about 38% of people who experienced at least two migraines a month reported experiencing exercise-triggered migraine attacks. The study found that high-intensity exercise was the most common type of activity reported by participants. However, the study did not explore whether substituting other types of activities could reduce the frequency of these migraines.

Some people may experience exercise-induced headaches or exertional headaches while engaging in physical activities. Exercise is designed to elevate heart rate and blood pressure, contributing to its effects.

These headaches are distinct from other migraines as they are typically triggered by exercise and occur during or after exertion. They can persist for varying durations ranging from as little as five minutes up to two days, and they are more prevalent in hot climates or at higher elevations.

It's important to rule out any medical conditions that could be causing these types of headaches.

For these people, I would recommend staying active with gentle movements, like walking, and not during the peak of a migraine attack but between episodes

Is It Safe to Work Out While You Have a Migraine?

The answer varies depending on circumstances, treatment plans, and medical advice. Generally, if the migraine pain is intense, it is advisable to postpone your exercise plans.

If you're having headaches while working out, it's a good idea to check in with a doctor to make sure there aren't any health issues that could be causing these headaches. If your headaches get worse when you exercise, it is recommended to keep an eye on your blood pressure during and after physical activity. This is crucial because untreated high blood pressure can show its symptoms when you're exercising, and it's something to review with your health care professional or a trained exercise specialist.

Exercising Safely

To exercise safely and avoid headaches, it's necessary to take precautions during and after physical activity. Here are some helpful tips to keep yourself safe and healthy while working out.

- **Fuel your body:** For those who are prone to experiencing an excessive drop in blood sugar during exercise, have a snack or light meal that includes carbohydrates, protein, and fats one to four hours before you exercise. For instance, consider having Greek yogurt with berries or a peanut butter and banana sandwich. Also, remember to have a meal with carbs and protein after your workout.

- **Stay hydrated:** Drinking water before, during, and after your workout is essential for overall well-being and headache prevention. If you're doing endurance activities lasting more than an hour, think about hydrating with a drink with added minerals.

- **Preparation and recovery:** Before you start exercising, warm up your body for at least three to five minutes with activities like walking or dynamic stretching. After your workout session, spend around five minutes doing stretches to help your heart rate and blood pressure return to normal.

- **Choose your exercises carefully:** Be mindful of the activities you engage in as some may be more likely than others to trigger headaches. Engaging in activities such as cycling, yoga, jogging, walking, and stretching has been associated with a reduction in the frequency of migraine episodes per monthly cycle.

Let's explore aerobic exercise guidelines that will help you before we close this chapter. Additionally in the next chapter, we will examine the benefits of yoga stretching routines and other physical exercises aimed at alleviating pain and stress to provide you with a strategy for managing your headaches through exercise.

Exercise for Migraines: Guidelines and Recommendations

Here are some important tips on how to include exercise in your routine, to help you handle your migraines better.

Aerobic Exercise Guidelines

- **Frequency:** Try to engage in moderate-level activity for about 2.5 to 5 hours per week, or opt for vigorous-intensity aerobic exercises for around 1.25 to 2.5 hours weekly (U.S. Department of Health and Human Services, 2023).

- **Intensity:** Aerobic workouts can range from intensity, from gentle walking to more vigorous activities such as running or jogging.

- **Duration:** Try to incorporate this activity into your routine, aiming to do it on most days.

Additional Recommendations

As mentioned above, regular physical activity has been shown to reduce the frequency and intensity of migraines in some individuals. Exercise can also help improve mood, reduce stress levels, and promote overall well-being, all of which can be beneficial for migraine management.

In addition to aerobic exercise, include balance and stretching activities to enhance flexibility and muscle-strengthening workouts targeting large muscle groups two or more times a week. The World Health Organization (WHO, 2011) recommends that aerobic activity should be done in sessions of 10 minutes before taking a break, and further recommends the same duration of weekly aerobic activities and strength exercises for major muscle groups twice weekly.

Strength training goes beyond simply developing muscles; it's about boosting your overall health. When you regularly do strength exercises, you're not only getting stronger but also increasing your lean muscle mass. This muscle boost is key for improving your metabolic health, which we'll dive into more in Chapter 8 of this book.

For older adults, the recommendation is at least 2.5 hours of moderate-intensity aerobic exercise, and 2 days of muscle-strengthening per week (U.S. Department of Health and Human Services, 2023). If you have been diagnosed with other chronic conditions, it's best to first consult with your doctor.

Before starting any exercise program, especially if you have health issues, consult with your doctor. Begin with small, manageable activities and gradually increase the intensity and duration as you build your fitness level. Focus on activities you enjoy, such as walking, cycling, or dancing, to make exercise more enjoyable and sustainable.

Moderate vs. High-Intensity Exercise

Moderate-intensity exercise allows you to maintain a conversation during the activity, while high-intensity exercise is more challenging and may only allow for a few words before you need to catch your breath.

High-intensity interval training (HIIT) is a great way to improve cardiovascular fitness in a short amount of time, but be careful not to overdo it. It's best to avoid during migraine attacks.

Duration and Intensity

Engaging in short bursts of physical activity throughout the day can lead to substantial improvements in health. Aim for a heart rate of around 60% of your maximum heart rate for moderate-intensity exercise and up to 80–90% for high-intensity exercise, depending on your fitness level (Harvard Health Publishing, 2023).

Examples of Aerobic Exercises

Aerobics, walking, cycling, hiking, dancing, rowing, and gardening are all excellent forms of aerobic exercise. Breaking up your aerobic workouts into 10-minute sessions throughout the day can yield significant cardiovascular benefits.

In conclusion, regular aerobic exercise, along with other types of physical activity, can be beneficial for persons with migraines. Consult with your healthcare provider before starting any new exercise program, and remember to start slowly and increase the intensity and duration gradually as you become more comfortable.

Yoga and Other Somatic Exercises

Managing stress is an important precautionary measure to curb migraines. When you participate in mind-body exercises like yoga and other somatic exercises like Pilates, tai chi, and daily stretching, you'll help to reduce your migraines and tension headaches by releasing chronic muscle tightness.

As part of a holistic healthcare approach, doing these mindful movement practices will promote your wellness in many different ways.

Yoga has been recognized to help in treating migraines and reducing their frequency and intensity. It helps relieve migraines by relaxing contracted muscles, promoting a sense of calm, and enhancing blood circulation. Additionally, when yoga is performed as a mindful movement practice, it offers the added benefits of mindfulness. This aspect of yoga encourages present-moment awareness, which can help reduce stress and improve overall well-being—both of which help with migraine management.

Some yoga positions are beneficial for alleviating tension in your neck, shoulders, and back, areas often affected by migraines. When combined with deep breathing techniques (called pranayama), they can have help decrease stress by calming your ANS, and thus avoiding migraines. We will discuss yoga, meditation, and deep breathing in more detail in the next chapter. First, let's have a look at some basic somatic exercises for migraine relief.

Somatic Exercises for Migraine Relief

Somatic exercises can ease migraines and headaches by helping you relax, lower your stress, and boost your overall well-being. Here are a few somatic exercises to try:

- **Body scan meditation:** Lie down and check your body for any tension or stress, focusing on one area at a time. Take a moment to feel if there's any tightness. If you find any, try to let go of the tension and give that body part a little relaxation. And remember, just like your head, your toes need a break sometimes, too!

- **Grounding:** Use the 5-4-3-2-1 coping method. Look around and name five things you see, touch four things, listen for three sounds, smell two scents, and taste one thing.

- **Self-soothing butterfly breathing:** Take a deep breath through your nose and gently tap your hands on your arms one after the other. Embrace the fluttery calmness!

- **Prolonged exhale-focused breathing:** Certain breathing techniques that emphasize the exhale can help rebalance your ANS, which regulates many automatic bodily functions like heart rate, digestion, and even migraine processes. During a migraine attack, the sympathetic "fight-or-flight" side of the ANS goes into overdrive. Prolonged exhalations can stimulate the parasympathetic "rest-and-digest" system to counteract this.

  - **The 4-3-7 breathing method:** Inhale through your nose for a count of 4, hold for 3 seconds, then exhale slowly for a count of 7. The extended exhale helps activate your vagus nerve, which runs from your brainstem through the body, distributing parasympathetic signals.

  - **Cyclic sighing breathing:** Start with a long, slow inhale through your nose. Then sigh out an audible exhale, consciously pushing out all the air. Aim for longer exhales compared to your inhaling. Repeat this inhale-sigh-exhale cycle for a few minutes. The sigh exhalations tap into your natural physiological sigh mechanism to trigger nervous system relaxation.

Making these exercises a regular habit can help counterbalance migraine-linked autonomic dysregulation over time. Even a few cycles during an attack may provide relief by activating your migraine-calming parasympathetic pathways. With practice, these conscious techniques can become an invaluable mindful tool in your migraine management toolkit.

We will cover more about yoga and breathwork in Chapter 5.

Exercise and Physical Activity: Implementation

Based on what we've discussed in this chapter, here are some practical tips to help you implement movement into your routine.

- **Regular aerobic exercise:** Engage in regular aerobic exercise like walking, cycling, swimming, or light jogging. Aerobic activity can help reduce migraine frequency and severity.

- **Strengthening exercises:** Incorporate strengthening exercises like weight training or bodyweight exercises into your routine. Building muscle strength can improve posture and reduce muscle tension.

- **Mind-body practices:** Try mind-body practices like yoga, Pilates, or tai chi, which combine physical movements with breath work and mindfulness.

- **Activity tracking apps:** Use apps and wearable devices to track your exercise levels, set goals, and stay motivated.

- **Workout videos/classes:** Take advantage of online workout videos or classes for guided exercise sessions.

Maintaining a consistent exercise routine incorporating a variety of aerobic, strength training, and mind-body activities can be an effective strategy for migraine management.

Key Takeaways

- **Exercise and migraines:** Don't think you have to avoid exercise just because you get migraines. With some smart strategies, being physically active can actually help manage your symptoms.

- **Low-impact aerobic exercises:** Walking, cycling, and swimming tend to be migraine-friendly options that can reduce attack frequency and severity over time.

- **High-intensity workouts:** While vigorous workouts may trigger migraines for some people, don't write off this kind of exercise altogether. Ease into your exercise routine gradually to find your personal limits.

- **Respecting your body's signals:** During a migraine attack, listen to your body. Pushing through intense exercise could potentially make things worse, so rest up and hydrate instead.

- **Yoga, stretching, and mind-body practices:** These are secret weapons for mellowing out muscle tension and quieting that inner-mind chatter that often accompanies migraines.

- **A consistent workout routine:** This isn't just about migraines—it's an investment in your overall physical and mental well-being, potentially boosting your resilience.

- **Be patient and keep notes:** Document what types of exercise help or aggravate your migraines. It may take some experimenting, but you can find that magical combo of activities to enhance your quality of life.

The key is tuning in to your body's signals, keeping an open mind, and crafting an exercise approach that works for you, not against you, in your migraine journey. Don't let migraines stop you from moving!

*****

In the next chapter, we'll explore the fascinating connection between your gut and your brain, and how this relationship impacts your overall health and well-being.

Chapter 4:
The Relationship Between Your Gut and Brain

Have you ever felt like your gut and brain are somehow connected? Well, it turns out they are—and this connection is especially important when it comes to migraines.

Think of your gut and brain like two best friends who are always chatting with each other. They use things like chemicals called neurotransmitters, the bacteria in your gut, and even stress hormones to communicate back and forth. Pretty cool, right?

Migraineurs often also experience gastrointestinal issues like diarrhea, constipation, heartburn, irritable bowel syndrome (IBS), stomach infections, inflammatory bowel disease, or celiac disease. These gut-related problems suggest a potential link between migraine and digestive system dysfunction, implying that when the gut is not functioning optimally, the brain may also be affected (Spekker & Nagy-Grócz, 2023).

And get this—some research suggests that taking probiotics (the good bacteria that keep your gut healthy) might help reduce how often you get migraines and how bad they are (Spekker & Nagy-Grócz, 2023). It's like giving your gut buddy a little reinforcement to help it communicate better with your brain buddy.

Understanding this close friendship between your gut and brain can help you find better ways to treat and manage your migraines. By figuring out how to keep that line of communication running smoothly, we might even be able to develop new strategies to prevent or reduce those painful migraine attacks.

So the next time you have a migraine, remember that it's not just your brain feeling out of order—your gut might be playing a role, too. Taking care of both of these buddies could be your key to feeling better.

The Gut Microbiome and Migraines

You've probably heard about all those tiny bacteria living in your gut—we're talking trillions of them! Well, it turns out that having the right balance of these microscopic creatures is super important, especially when it comes to migraines.

See, when the mixture of bacteria gets out of line, it's like having a bunch of unruly houseguests that start causing trouble. This imbalance, called dysbiosis, has been linked to more frequent and severe migraine attacks.

Certain species of bacteria can produce inflammatory molecules that might trigger migraines in some people, and other types of bacteria can influence the levels of brain chemicals called neurotransmitters. As you might have guessed, when those get out of balance, migraines can come knocking at your door.

The research on this is pretty fascinating. Studies have found that the gut microbiome (the mix of all those bacteria) in people with migraines is quite different from those who don't get migraines (Spekker & Nagy-Grócz, 2023). It's like their gut is housing a completely different set of tiny tenants!

So if your gut microbiome is all out of sorts, it could be setting you up for more migraines. Taking care of this internal ecosystem is an important way to keep your head from pounding.

Now, don't go evicting all your gut bacteria just yet! The goal is to get them living in a balanced, harmonious community again. We'll talk about how to do that a little later. But first, let's look at another piece of this gut-brain puzzle.

The Role of Diet and Probiotics

Okay, so now that we know just how important it is to have a balanced gut microbiome, let's talk about what you can eat to keep those tiny tenants happy!

Nutritious Foods Support a Healthy Gut Environment

The foods you choose to eat have a huge impact on the types of bacteria that set up camp in your gut. You want to provide the good stuff that lets the beneficial bacteria thrive, rather than the other way around.

Some foods act like fertilizer (prebiotics) for the fiber-munching, inflammation-reducing bacteria. Things like fruits, veggies, whole grains, and legumes are buffets for the good guys. They're jam-packed with fiber that keeps these microbes well-fed and doing their jobs properly.

But here's the best part—you can help reinforce the good bacteria's ranks by consuming prebiotics and probiotics, which are like shipping in some extra well-behaved houseguests to join the party in your gut. Pre- and probiotics may come in supplement form, and you can also get them from fermented foods like yogurt, kefir, sauerkraut, and kimchi.

On the flip side, a diet heavy in processed foods, fried stuff, added sugars, and saturated fats can enable the growth of inflammatory, troublemaking bacteria. We're talking about the rowdy ones that might trigger migraines.

So load up on those fruits, veggies, fiber, and probiotic-rich foods to support the growth of beneficial bacteria and reduce migraines. Your gut buddies will be happy, which means your brain buddy is more likely to stay happy too!

Potential Benefits of Probiotics for Reducing Migraines

Probiotics present an opportunity for developing healthy bacteria. Let's explore the potential benefits of probiotic supplementation for restoring your gut microbiome balance and, as a result, reducing your migraine frequency.

Taking probiotic supplements may help reduce the number of migraine attacks you experience. A study looked at the effects of a probiotic containing *Lactobacillus* and *Bifidobacterium* strains on episodic migraine patients. After eight weeks of supplementation, the probiotic group suffered significantly fewer migraine days compared to the placebo group (Gao et al., 2020).

Another study found that a multi-strain probiotic supplement was able to reduce the frequency, severity, and disability of migraine attacks in chronic migraine patients after 10 weeks of use. The researchers attributed this to the probiotics helping restore gut microbiome equilibrium (Dimidi et al., 2019).

Adding Probiotic-Rich Foods to Your Diet

Remember, a happier gut leads to a happier you! Here are some practical tips to easily incorporate probiotic-rich foods into your diet:

Yogurt

- If possible, avoid yogurts with artificial sweeteners or added sugars.

- Consider yogurts that say "contains live and active cultures." Greek and Icelandic yogurts often have more probiotic strains.

- Top with granola, nuts, or seeds, and fresh fruit for a healthy breakfast.

- Use it as a base for dips, dressings, or smoothies.

- Replace things like sour cream or mayonnaise with plain yogurt in recipes.

Kefir

- This fermented dairy drink has a tart, refreshing flavor similar to drinkable yogurt.

- Have a glass of plain kefir in the morning or use it in smoothies. Add some frozen fruit to the smoothie for flavor.

- Use kefir as the liquid in pancake or waffle batter recipes.

- Prepare it as a frozen treat (almost like ice cream). You could serve it with some berry sauce or, for a healthier option, add some fruit (either fresh or frozen) on top.

Kimchi

- This Korean staple is loaded with lactic acid bacteria from fermentation.

- Use it as a flavorful topping for rice bowls, stir-fries, or eggs.

- Add a spoonful to soups or stews after you're done cooking for a probiotic boost.

- Try vegan kimchi if you avoid eating fish.

Sauerkraut

- Look for refrigerated sauerkraut without vinegar added to get live probiotics.

- Add a scoop on top of salads, sandwiches, burgers, or avocado toast.

- Incorporate it into egg or tuna salad.

- Sauté it with some vegetables and protein for a quick, probiotic-packed meal.

Other Tips

- Start slow if these foods are new to your diet and build up gradually.

- Buy smaller amounts more frequently to ensure maximum freshness.

- Make your own probiotic-rich foods at home to control ingredients.

Getting creative with incorporating these probiotic powerhouses can make it easy to achieve healthy microbiome restoration!

Gut Permeability and Inflammation

Your intestines have an incredibly important job—acting as a gatekeeper to let nutrients in while keeping harmful substances out. The gut lining forms a selective barrier, only allowing properly digested food particles and other beneficial compounds to pass into the bloodstream.

However, sometimes this barrier gets a bit too porous or "leaky." This condition, known as increased intestinal permeability or "leaky gut," allows larger molecules and toxins to slip through the gut lining into the body where they don't belong.

Leaky gut is thought to be caused by factors like poor diet, chronic stress, bacterial imbalance, and certain medications that can damage the delicate gut lining over time.

When these larger molecules escape into the bloodstream, the body recognizes them as foreign invaders and mounts an inflammatory response to attack them. This results in widespread inflammation throughout the body.

Inflammation is a normal immune process in small doses, but chronic inflammation is a major driver of many health concerns like autoimmune conditions, neurological disorders, and even migraines.

In fact, studies have found that migraine sufferers tend to have higher levels of certain inflammatory markers in their blood compared to non-migraineurs. This systemic inflammation could potentially contribute to the neuroinflammation thought to trigger migraine attacks (Edvinsson et al., 2019).

By allowing inflammatory compounds through the gut lining and into circulation, a leaky gut could be setting the stage for the widespread inflammation and neuroinflammation involved in migraine pathogenesis. Maintaining a healthy, strict gut barrier is important for migraine management by preventing the influx of inflammatory triggers from a permeable intestinal lining.

We've talked about how a "leaky gut" allows the wrong kinds of molecules to escape from the intestines into the body. Well, this breach in the gut barrier can set off an inflammatory red alert!

It's like the gut is the spark that sets off an inflammatory wildfire, which then rages its way up to your head, leaving you with a fierce migraine in its wake. By keeping that gut lining strong and sealed up tight, you can help prevent inflammatory molecules from crossing over in the first place. This lowers the overall inflammation levels coursing through your body and brain.

With less out-of-control inflammation mucking up the works, your migraine attacks might occur less frequently or feel less intense. It's all about smothering those inflammatory sparks before they can ignite into searing migraines.

Taking steps to heal a leaky gut and calm widespread inflammation could be a game-changer for preventing migraines at their source. Find out more on how to do that below!

How to Improve Your Gut Integrity

There are some great ways to help improve gut integrity and seal up your intestinal lining. Let's explore some tips.

Food Fixes

Eating the right foods and consuming nutritious drinks are crucial for your gut health.

- Avoid inflammatory foods that can further damage the gut like processed meats, fried foods, sugar, refined carbs, and anything you're allergic to. Also, steer clear of triggering foods if you are glucose or lactose intolerant.

- Load up on anti-inflammatory foods like fatty fish, turmeric, ginger, leafy greens, berries, olive oil, and bone broth.

- Get plenty of prebiotic fiber from veggies, fruits, legumes, and whole grains. Fiber nourishes the good bacteria in your gut, promoting a healthy digestive system.

- Replace sugary drinks and sodas with water and herbal teas.

- Avoid dietary factors like MSG (monosodium glutamate), caffeine, and alcohol that can worsen migraines.

- Special diets, such as the ketogenic and low-glycemic-index diets, may be effective in reducing how often and how severe your migraines are. Consider following a specific eating plan tailored to your needs. It's essential to consult with a healthcare professional before making significant changes to your diet to ensure it aligns with your health goals.

Supplement Helpers

In addition to a healthy diet, certain supplements can support gut healing and integrity.

- L-glutamine powder can help rebuild and repair the intestinal lining.

- Collagen supplements provide gut-healing amino acids.

- Zinc L-carnosine supports and strengthens gut defenses.

- Deglycyrrhizinated licorice soothes and coats the gut lining.

- Marshmallow root contains mucilage that protects intestinal walls.

- Probiotic supplements reintroduce beneficial bacteria.

Lifestyle Upgrades

- Manage stress through meditation, deep breathing, and yoga, as chronic stress wears on the gut.

- Get enough sleep and allow time for your gut to rest and restore overnight.

- Move your body regularly with mild exercise like brisk walks or taking the stairs instead of the elevator.

- Ensuring proper hydration, especially when consuming fiber-rich foods, supports your gut's function and prevents digestive issues.

The goal is to minimize attacks on your gut while providing the right building blocks to strengthen your intestinal barrier. With a sturdy gut lining, fewer inflammatory compounds can slip through and trigger migraines.

Wrapping Up

Improving your gut integrity is a journey that requires attention to both diet and lifestyle factors. By making conscious choices to support your gut health through nourishing foods, targeted supplements, and healthy habits, you can enhance your gut lining and reduce the likelihood of inflammatory compounds causing migraines. Experimenting with different approaches and being patient with your body's healing process can lead to long-term benefits for your gut health and overall well-being.

Disturbances in Gut-Brain Pathways and Migraines

Let's explore the various pathways that allow your gut and brain to communicate bi-directionally—and some ways this communication can be impeded.

Out-of-Whack Neurotransmitters

Believe it or not, your gut produces a ton of the same neurotransmitters that your brain uses to send signals. Compounds such as dopamine, GABA, serotonin, and glutamate are produced in the gut. These chemicals can then enter the bloodstream and travel right up to the brain, impacting mood, pain perception, and bodily processes. An imbalance of these gut neurotransmitters could potentially contribute to migraine episodes. For example, low levels of serotonin have been linked to gut issues like IBS as well as an increased risk of migraines.

Immune Molecule Messengers: Inflammatory Overload

The gut and brain are constantly swapping important immune molecules and cellular messages back and forth, which means inflammatory molecules like cytokines produced in the gut can instigate inflammation in the brain and central nervous system. Conversely, the brain's inflammatory signals can disrupt the gut microbiome and intestinal lining. This two-way street of immune communication can perpetuate neurological and gut conditions.

A leaky or permeable gut allows inflammatory molecules and particles to enter the bloodstream. This chronic inflammation can then make its way to the brain, causing neuroinflammation.

Triggers for Migraines

When the body's natural defense system reacts to things that are harmful, it can lead to migraines. For example, if someone is feeling a lot of stress, their body might react by causing inflammation, which can affect how different parts of your brain work.

One way this happens is through the trigeminal network, which is like a communication system in the brain that sends signals about pain. When this network is activated, it can make you more sensitive to pain, which can lead to migraines.

Your body's signaling system can also experience disruption, impacting the transmission of messages between different parts of your brain and body. If the neurotransmitters, which are like messengers in your brain, are not working correctly, it can lead to problems like migraines.

Vagus Nerve Miscommunication

The vagus nerve is the superhighway between the gut and brain. This long nerve runs from the brainstem down through the abdomen, allowing bi-directional communication. Gut bacteria can send signals through the vagus nerve to influence brain function, and the brain can transmit responses back down the vagus to modulate gut movement, nutrient absorption, and immunity.

Gut-Hormone Havoc

The gut produces and secretes dozens of hormones that can then travel through the body and impact the brain. Gut hormones like ghrelin, leptin, cholecystokinin, and peptide YY help manage hunger, inflammation levels, mood, and more. These chemical messengers from the gut provide another communication pathway to influence neurological processes.

So, in many ways, your gut is almost like your second brain, sending and receiving constant messages! Disruptions in any of these intricate signaling pathways could contribute to gut-based migraine triggers. Maintaining a healthy dialogue between these two intelligent systems is key for prevention.

Gut disorders and microbiome dysbiosis can disrupt the normal production of appetitive hormones like ghrelin, leptin, and others. These hormonal imbalances emerging from gut issues could influence migraine pathways by increasing neuroinflammation, altering pain perception, and affecting neurotransmitters.

Essentially, all these gut-brain communication channels are closely interlinked. So if there are problems in the gut like leaky gut, bacterial overgrowths, inflammation, and others, it can cause systemic disturbances in neurotransmitters, immune molecules, vagus nerve signals, and hormones.

Addressing the root gut imbalances could help restore normal cross-talk between the gut and brain. This may allow for improved migraine prevention and management by eliminating migraine triggers at their source.

Stress and the Mind-Body Connection

The mind-body connection between emotional stress and both gut health and migraine susceptibility is fascinating. Lifestyle habits such as stress, not getting enough sleep, and lack of physical activity can mess up the balance of the good bacteria in your gut and make migraines worse. Let's explore this in more detail.

The Impact of Emotional Stress on Gut Health and Migraines

At the core of this mind-body link is the brain-gut axis we've been discussing—that bi-directional superhighway between our gut and our brain. When we experience high levels of emotional or psychological stress, it triggers the release of hormones and neurotransmitters that can directly impact the gut.

Stress causes an increase in cortisol, the body's main stress hormone. While cortisol is helpful for providing energy boosts in small doses, chronic high levels can lead to gut inflammation, increased permeability (leaky gut), and imbalances in gut bacteria.

Stress also prompts the brain to send signals down the vagus nerve to the gut. This can alter gut motility, reduce blood flow and nutrient absorption, and disrupt the gut-brain communication highway.

The result? Gut issues like indigestion, diarrhea, constipation, nausea, and flares of conditions like IBS or IBD can occur during stressful periods. And as we know, an unhappy, inflamed gut can then send molecular messages back up to the brain, contributing to migraine pathogenesis.

But it's not just the gut that gets disrupted—stress can prime the brain for migraines through other mechanisms, too. It depletes serotonin, which can trigger migraines, as well as increases muscle tension in your head or neck, disrupts your sleep, and lowers your pain threshold.

This creates the perfect storm for migraines to develop—a sensitized, primed brain combined with an irritated, leaky gut all stemming from excessive stress levels. However, proven mind-body techniques like meditation, deep breathing, yoga, and cognitive behavioral therapy can help reinforce the communication pathways and counteract these physiological stress effects.

Promote your gut health by learning to calm your mind. This will help reduce whole-body inflammation and lower your susceptibility to migraines, making the mind-body connection a powerful tool against pesky migraine attacks.

Key Takeaways

- **The gut-brain link:** Your gut and brain are linked, communicating through a pathway called the gut-brain axis. This relationship plays a big role in many aspects of your health, including how your migraines develop.

- **Gut health and migraines:** Imbalances in the gut's bacteria and inflammation can contribute to migraines, affecting how often you get them and how severe they are.

- **Eating for your gut:** Changing your diet, like cutting back on processed foods and eating more high-fiber foods can help keep your gut healthy and might reduce how often you get migraines.

- **Probiotics and supplements:** Taking probiotics and certain supplements could ease migraine symptoms by keeping your gut healthy.

- **Stress and gut health:** Managing stress through practices like yoga, mindfulness, and relaxation can support your gut health, possibly reducing the severity and frequency of your migraines.

- **A whole-person approach:** Taking care of your gut and brain health together, as part of a bigger picture of your overall health, can be really helpful in managing migraines and feeling better overall.

Our gut microbiome, that teeming society of microbes residing in our intestines, fundamentally shapes not just our digestive health, but our brain health and susceptibility to migraine attacks.

By nurturing a flourishing inner garden through a nutrient-dense diet, we can cultivate the right microbial balance to reduce inflammation, optimize neurotransmitter production, and keep the gut-brain communication highways clear of debris. Although the journey is an intensely personal one, the path starts by listening to your body's innate wisdom and treating your gut as the important player it truly is.

*****

In the next chapter, we will look at combining your gut health strategies with other holistic practices like meditation, movement, and quality sleep, because taking exquisite care of your gut may be the missing piece that helps you finally break free from migraine's relentless grip.

Chapter 5:
Stress Management

If you just can't seem to find lasting migraine relief from conventional medications and treatments, you're not alone! A significant number of migraine warriors have started exploring alternatives outside of the mainstream medical world.

We're talking about things like meditation, mindfulness practices, and acupuncture, or trying out natural herbal remedies and supplements. A social media survey shows that up to a whopping 90% of migraine patients in the United States have given these holistic approaches a try (Kuruvilla et al., 2021).

So why the surge in alternative treatments? For many, it's because traditional medicine and therapies either haven't worked for them or caused nasty side effects. Others simply haven't tried them yet, hoping to find more natural, side-effect-free ways to keep migraines at bay.

It's important to acknowledge that these alternative migraine treatments are not a complete replacement for mainstream therapies. They're meant to be used in combination as a complementary approach (Kuruvilla, 2018).

You can consider the use of complementary therapies before using prescription medicine, or to support the use of medicine—incorporate meditation, acupuncture, or nutraceuticals as boosters to the overall treatment plan.

The goal is to find that perfect, personalized recipe that works for your body and brain. For some, that might mean meditating to reduce migraine triggers. For others, it could be acupuncture sessions or specific vitamin supplements.

At the end of the day, managing migraines is already difficult enough. If safe, natural alternatives can provide extra relief when combined with medical treatments, it's definitely worth exploring. Don't be afraid to get creative and find what works best for you. Also, do discuss these with your doctor.

Mind-Body Practices to Reduce Stress

Employing mind-body practices can help reduce your stress level and its negative impacts on both your gut health and susceptibility to migraines. Let's discuss some of these approaches.

Meditation

Taking time to meditate, even just 10 to 15 minutes per day, can work wonders. Practices like mindfulness meditation, breath focus, and body scans help calm the mind, lower cortisol and adrenaline levels, and promote feelings of relaxation. This can translate to reduced gut inflammation and a reduced prevalence of migraines (Wells et al., 2014).

Migraine Relief: A Mindful Meditation Recipe

Let me walk you through a simple yet powerful meditation "recipe" that can be great for migraine management.

- First, find a quiet, comfortable space where you can relax without distractions for 10 to 15 minutes. You can sit on a cushion or in a chair with your feet securely on the ground. Gently close your eyes or keep them slightly open and unfocused.

- Start by bringing your attention to your breathing. Inhale slowly through your nose, allowing your belly to expand. Then exhale fully. Don't force it, just breathe naturally. As you exhale, envision all tension dissipating from your body.

- As you continue these deep, diaphragmatic breaths, you can silently repeat a soothing mantra like "I am calm" or "I am at peace." This anchors your mind to the present moment.

- Now, direct your focus inward by doing a gentle body scan. Notice any areas of tightness or tension, maybe in your shoulders, jaw, or temples—common migraine hot spots. Consciously breathe into these areas, imagining them becoming more relaxed with each exhalation.

- You can also visualize healing energy or light flowing to any area of pain or discomfort in your head and neck. Imagine the tension melting away, softening your face, and smoothing out any creases on your forehead.

- If your mind begins to drift (it happens!), avoid self-judgment. Simply acknowledge the thought and return your attention to your breath.

- After 10 to 15 minutes of this conscious breathing, body awareness, and visualization, you can gently open your eyes and carry that sense of serenity with you as you resume your day.

The key is to create a small oasis of calm amid the migraine storm. With regular practice, meditation strengthens mind-body connections vital for migraine relief. Customize your meditation further by adding mantras, imagery, or any elements that resonate with you!

Gut-Directed Hypnotherapy

This mind-body therapy is a fascinating complementary therapy that utilizes hypnosis scripts specifically designed to target the gut-brain connection. The premise involves using hypnotic suggestions and guided imagery to directly influence the gut-brain axis, which plays a crucial role in migraine pathogenesis. Visual imagery helps relax and heal gut function while alleviating stress responses in the brain, essentially giving the gut-brain communication pathway a hypnotic tune-up. In the Bonus chapter, valuable resources like guided imagery apps will be explored.

During a typical session, you'll work with a certified hypnotherapist. They'll guide you into a deeply relaxed, trance-like state of focused attention.

While in this heightened state of awareness, the therapist will suggest multi-sensory visualizations designed to communicate with your subconscious mind. The imagery will be specifically crafted to help relax and heal your gut function.

For example, they might guide you to envision your gut as a beautiful, peaceful garden where healthy plant life (representing balanced gut microbes) can thrive. Or see your intestinal walls as a flexible, semi-permeable boundary that keeps out toxic invaders.

The suggestions work to reprogram your gut-brain signals at a subconscious level. Releasing physical tension, boosting blood flow, optimizing nutrient absorption, and restoring gastrointestinal motility patterns.

While your gut is being "reprogrammed," the hypnotherapist will also introduce language to dial down excessive stress responses in the brain. Dampening the flames of inflammation, relaxing tense muscle fibers, and interrupting your hyper-vigilant, pain-focused brain state.

It's like a hypnotic reboot for your gut-brain superhighway, relieving the traffic jams, construction zones, and glitches in communication that contribute to migraines.

Typically, you'd go through a series of these gut-directed hypnotherapy sessions, building on the subconscious programming each time. The idea is to forge new neural pathways for healthy gut-brain interaction.

Many find it to be a profoundly relaxing and cathartic experience, but it does require working with a skilled professional. With regular practice, it's an innovative way to naturally realign your gut-brain balance.

Yoga Poses For Stress-Induced Migraines

This section builds on what we covered in Chapter 3 about yoga and breathwork. Yoga usually involves mindfulness and relaxation methods like meditation that aid in reducing stress—an identified trigger for many migraine attacks. The practice of yoga has potential benefits as it may help decrease sympathetic overactivity while supporting parasympathetic dominance, as well as regulating autonomic nervous system activity. All of these factors could contribute toward preventing migraines from occurring.

However, people with migraines need to practice yoga carefully, maybe even with someone guiding them. This is important especially when a person has an active migraine episode because they have to choose postures and techniques that won't worsen their symptoms.

The combination of gentle movement, deep breathing, and mindfulness in yoga is a powerful stress-buster. Certain poses can also provide a massage for the vagus nerve to support good gut-brain communication.

Yoga may lessen tension headache occurrence, duration, and pain severity (Anheyer et al., 2020), though more research is needed to confirm yoga as a useful treatment for migraines. Nevertheless, a more recent study suggests that managing migraines with stress management using mindfulness can be helpful (Wells et al., 2021). Previous research has also revealed that combining standard treatments with yoga exercises can effectively lower the incidence and intensity of migraine attacks (Kisan et al., 2014).

When stress starts brewing up a migraine storm, certain yoga poses can be incredibly calming for both your body and mind. It's like giving your nervous system a full-body "ahhhh" to interrupt that headache-inducing tension. Let's look at some yoga techniques to reduce your stress (Mandriota, 2022).

Child's Pose

This is one of my go-to's when I need a reset. Kneel with your big toes closely knit and your knees spread apart. Then walk your hands out in front of you and allow your torso to melt toward your thighs. Let your forehead come to rest on the mat if possible. Breathe deeply into the backbend as you surrender tension. If helpful, you can hold your head and arms somewhat elevated, like on a chair.

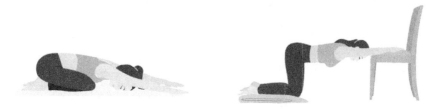

Cat and Cow Poses

To execute the cat pose, position yourself on all fours, ensuring your wrists are aligned under your shoulders and your knees are beneath your hips. Inhale deeply, and as you exhale, round your back up toward the ceiling. Lower your chin into your chest and draw your belly button toward your spine. The position should resemble the shape of a cat stretching its back. Hold this pose for a few breaths, engaging your abdominal muscles and feeling the stretch along your back and shoulders.

From the cat pose, inhale and drop your belly toward the floor, simultaneously lifting your head and tailbone toward the ceiling. Your body should form an inverted "U" shape, with your gaze directed upward. This position mimics the stance of a cow naturally arching its back. As you breathe out, return to the cat pose, repeating this easy movement in sync with your breath. This gentle spinal flexion and extension can help alleviate tension in your neck and back muscles, promoting relaxation and improving overall spinal mobility.

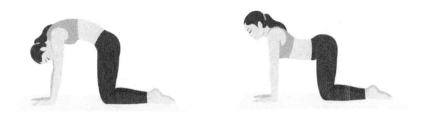

Feet-Up Pose

This versatile feet-up pose can help release tension and improve your sleep. It works well as part of a wind-down routine. Put your feet up against the wall, or on a chair with your knees bent. In this position, complete 10 cycles of slow long breaths with an exhale-focused breath. You may place one hand on your belly and the other hand on your chest to feel the movement of your breath.

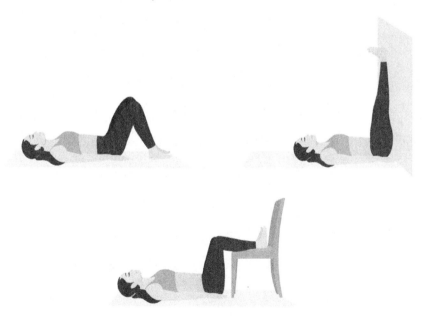

Savasana Pose

Sometimes, you just need to become one with your mat. Lie flat on your back, letting your arms and legs fall open. Close your eyes and focus on breathing fully into your belly as you consciously release any areas of tightness. This pose is ideal for quieting your mind.

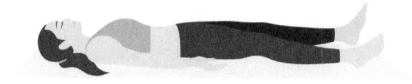

Adding Breathing to Your Poses

No matter which poses you explore, syncing them with some focused breathing is key. Try inhaling through your nose, and exhaling out for eight counts. This breathing, with a longer ratio of exhale compared to inhale, can amplify the stress-busting benefits.

You can even do a humming breath by making an "mmmm" sound on each exhale—it's an oddly satisfying vibration!

The most important thing is tuning in to what *your* body needs in that specific moment. Don't force any postures that cause strain. Carefully explore and keep returning to that conscious breathing. A little yoga therapy can be so centering when you feel a migraine start to percolate.

Deep Breathing

This is an easy and accessible way to quickly calm your mind and body. Practices like box or square breathing, 4-7-8 breathing, or diaphragmatic belly breathing can stimulate the vagus nerve, and lower your heart rate.

As a result it eases the "fight-or-flight" response of your ANS, reducing stress that contributes to migraines.

Breathing Exercises for Calming Migraines

When you feel those first rumblings of a migraine brewing, it's time to break out the breathwork. Simple breathing exercises can be a powerful tool for interrupting the cascading stress response that so often triggers or exacerbates head pain.

Diaphragmatic Belly Breathing

Before beginning breathing exercises, create a space where you feel calm and free from distractions. Decide what works best for you—maybe it's dimming the lights, lighting a candle, or finding a cozy corner to nestle into. Get yourself situated in a relaxed position, whether sitting or lying down.

Now bring your attention to your breath. Place one hand on your chest and the other on your belly. As you inhale through your nose, allow your abdomen to gently expand outward—like a balloon inflating. Picture your abdominal area as a sphere or cylinder, and feel the sensation of expansion radiating from your belly around to your lower back.

While your abdomen stretches with the inhalation, aim to keep your chest relatively relaxed, not rising significantly. Become aware of the full, three-dimensional expansion occurring in your abdominal cavity as you breathe in deeply through your nose. We're going for deep, diaphragmatic breaths here to oxygenate.

Once you have the hang of that belly breathing, you can explore different patterns.

Box Breathing

One I love is the "box breath" where you inhale for four counts, pause for four, exhale for four, pause for four—and repeat. It's like tracing the sides of a square with your breath.

You can also go with a more free-flowing approach. Simply breathe in through your nose, allowing your belly to expand. Then, slowly exhale through your nose, feeling your belly deflate. Don't force it—just find a natural, steady rhythm.

The longer you can sync up with your breath, the more you'll ease out of that contracted, pain-braced state. You may even enter a deeply relaxed, almost meditative zone where you disconnect from the painful sensations for a bit. Ahhh, sweet relief!

4-3-7 Breathing

When you feel a migraine attack brewing, one of the first things you could do is find a quiet spot to practice some 4-3-7 breathing. It's almost like a manual override for your respiratory system.

- Start by exhaling fully, getting all that stale air out of your lungs. Then breathe in slowly through your nose while mentally counting to four.

- Hold that breath for three counts. You can imagine trapping that fresh oxygen inside.

- Finally, exhale slowly through your nose for a count of seven, really trying to fully empty your lungs.

- The extended exhalation is key. It helps relieve any built-up muscle tension and flips your nervous system into rest-and-digest instead of fight-or-flight mode.

- Do rounds of 4-3-7 breathing for several minutes, focusing just on the counting pattern and flow of air.

There are other breathing patterns, such as the 4-7-8 technique (inhaling for four counts, holding for seven counts, and exhaling for eight counts). The key is to extend the exhalation longer than the inhalation, ideally aiming for an exhalation twice as long as the inhalation. Additionally, I recommend a brief pause (for example, three counts or more) before repeating the cycle.

The Physiological Sigh

This technique is very effective for lowering stress levels. First, take a full inhale, then an extra sniff at the end of the inhale. You can place you hands by the sides of your rib cage, to feel expand outward as you take in this extra breath. Then do a slow and long exhale.

It's a simple tool that short-circuits your body's stress response. It oxygenates your body while encouraging a profound state of relaxation and calm. Those tightened migraine circuits in your brain almost get a hard reset. It minimizes your pain and buys you time until other remedies can kick in.

The beauty is that you can practice these breathing exercises anywhere, anytime—at your desk, in the car, or even lying in a dark room with a cold compress when a full-blown attack hits. Even just 5 to 10 deep, conscious breaths can be migraine-quelling magic. Consider coupling it with aromatherapy, too, for extra relief.

Aim to make breathwork a regular practice. Just tune inward, sync up with that precious airflow, and let the restorative calm ripple through your mind and body. A little oxygen is one of nature's most potent migraine remedies!

Stress Management Techniques: Implementation

Here's a practical approach to implementing stress management techniques:

- **Stress diary:** Keep a diary to track your stress levels and migraine episodes. Note down stressful events or triggers to help you identify patterns.

- **Deep breathing:** Try using any of the breathwork techniques discussed in this chapter whenever you feel stressed or tense.

- **Progressive muscle relaxation:** Tense and then relax each muscle group in your body, starting from your toes and working up to your head. This can help release tension and reduce stress.

- **Mindfulness apps:** Use mindfulness meditation apps like Headspace, Calm, or Ten Percent Happier for guided meditation sessions. These apps can help you relax and manage stress anywhere, anytime. We also talk more about apps and resources to assist you on your wellness journey in the Bonus chapter.

- **Physical activity:** Engage in regular physical activity, such as walking, yoga, or dancing. Exercise can help reduce stress and improve your mood, which may help prevent migraines.

- **CBT techniques:** Learn cognitive-behavioral therapy (CBT) techniques to manage stress and change repetitive negative thinking. Online resources or self-help books can guide you through these techniques.

- **Support network:** Build your network of friends, family, or a support group for migraine sufferers to gain emotional solace and practical advice.

- **Professional help:** Consider seeking professional help from a therapist or counselor who specializes in stress management.

They can provide personalized strategies to help you cope with stress and reduce migraine frequency.

Key Takeaways

- **Mind-body approaches:** Practices like meditation, deep breathing, and yoga can help reduce stress levels and the associated migraine triggers.

- **Choose techniques that work best for you:** Specific meditation and breathing techniques like mindful breath focus, body scans, box breathing, and 4-3-7 or 4-7-8 breathing are recommended for calming the mind and body. Decide on which techniques to explore based on your personal requirements.

- **Explore yoga poses:** Certain yoga techniques like child's pose, cat/cow pose, and savasana can release tension and promote relaxation when done gently.

- **Gut-directed hypnotherapy**: Leverage guided imagery to improve your gut-brain communication and reduce migraine pathogenesis.

- **Practical stress management tips**: This includes keeping a stress diary, using mindfulness apps, exercising regularly, learning CBT techniques, building a support network, and seeking professional help if needed.

- **Reducing stress**: Through mind-body practices and lifestyle approaches you can reduce stress. This can be a powerful complement to medical migraine treatments.

*****

In the upcoming chapter, we'll explore the intricate relationship between female hormones and migraines, and what you can do to manage it effectively.

Chapter 6:
The Relationship Between Female Hormones and Migraines

If you're a woman who suffers from migraines, you're certainly not alone. In fact, migraine headaches tend to disproportionately affect women (Al-Hassany et al., 2020). But have you ever wondered about the underlying reason for this gender difference? In this chapter, we'll dive into the intricate relationship between female hormones and migraines.

Our hormones, those powerful chemical messengers, play a pivotal role in regulating countless bodily functions. For women, the ebb and flow of hormones like estrogen and progesterone orchestrate major life events such as menstruation, pregnancy, and menopause. However, their fluctuations can also have profound effects on the brain and its delicate neurochemistry.

As you'll discover, seemingly minor shifts in hormone levels can sometimes set off a complex cascade of events within your brain, altering the delicate balance of neurotransmitters and inflammatory responses. In some cases, this disruption can trigger the debilitating pain, nausea, and sensory hypersensitivity that characterize a migraine attack.

Throughout this chapter, we'll explore the fascinating interplay between specific hormonal changes and migraine susceptibility across different life stages. You'll gain insights into why migraines may worsen during certain times of the month, as well as how events like pregnancy and menopause can influence migraine patterns.

Understanding this relationship isn't just about satisfying curiosity about your next life phase; it's about empowerment. Armed with this knowledge, you can better anticipate potential migraine triggers and develop proactive strategies to manage hormonal fluctuations and minimize their impact on your migraine experiences.

So let's embark on this journey together, unraveling the connections between female hormones and migraines. By the end of this chapter, you'll have a deeper appreciation for the incredible complexity of the human body and be better equipped to navigate the unique challenges that come with being a migraine-prone woman.

The Link Between Hormones and Migraines

If you are a woman, you may be surprised to hear that at different ages, you may experience migraines differently, based on the hormonal phase you're in. Let's talk about the link between your hormones and migraines.

One in six women have migraines. You might be asking, "Why me? Why do I get migraines?" It's not your fault that you have migraines—they tend to run in families, even if your relative's headaches don't sound like yours. Migraine-prone brains are brains in a hypersensitive state, meaning that your brain is sensitive to your environment and can easily fire off a headache with the right combination of triggers.

Your Menstrual Cycle and Migraines

Have you ever noticed your blood sugar levels going haywire around that time of the month? Well, it's not just in your head! During the menstrual cycle, hormone fluctuations can actually mess with your body's ability to regulate blood sugar properly. Especially in the latter half of your cycle, you might experience more intense spikes and crashes in blood sugar levels, contributing to migraines.

For many women, one of the first telltale signs that hormones play a role in their migraines is the impact of their monthly menstrual cycle. As those hormone levels ebb and flow throughout the month, migraine patterns often follow suit.

There's a predictable relationship between migraines and menstruation for countless women. Some are especially prone to menstrual migraines, which give them painful headaches several days before or during their period when estrogen levels plummet (MacGregor et al., 2010). Others find their migraines tend to strike during the luteal phase after ovulation when progesterone levels take a nosedive (Calhoun, 2012).

While the exact mechanisms are complex, the dramatic hormone shifts before and during menstruation are thought by some researchers to trigger inflammatory pathways in the brain, making it easier for migraines to occur during this window (Pavlović et al., 2014).

This rollercoaster ride can be a major migraine trigger for some women. Rapid changes in blood sugar also cause inflammation and imbalances that make the problem worse. So if you're prone to menstrual migraines, keeping an eye on your blood sugar levels and trying to maintain stability through diet and exercise could help prevent those debilitating headaches. The tips described in Chapter 8, relating to metabolic factors, may be specifically helpful in this life stage.

Pregnancy and Postpartum Changes

The hormonal roller coaster continues during pregnancy and the postpartum period. Interestingly, many women enjoy a welcome reprieve from migraines during pregnancy. Approximately two-thirds of women, especially those with migraine without aura, experience a decrease in their migraines. This improvement usually happens in the second and third trimesters (Afridi, 2018). This is likely due to the high, sustained levels of estrogen that help stabilize brain chemistry (Sances et al., 2003).

However, the months immediately following childbirth often undo this respite. As hormones rapidly plummet to pre-pregnancy levels, the sudden shifts create a vulnerable period for postpartum migraines (Kvisvik et al., 2011). In addition, other postpartum factors like sleep deprivation, stress, and changing routines can compound the migraine risk. Breastfeeding can help provide protection against migraines, so this is another good reason to breastfeed, if you can (Calhoun, 2017).

The Menopausal Transition

During perimenopause, the period preceding menopause, there could also be various metabolic disturbances that could contribute to migraine. The techniques explained in the metabolic chapter may be useful during this period, so take notice when you get to Chapter 8.

The menopausal years present another significant hormonal shift for migraine management. As the ovaries gradually produce less estrogen and progesterone, women can experience erratic hormone fluctuations and an increased susceptibility to hormonally triggered migraines (Pavlović et al., 2017).

Every woman's experience is different. Some may sail through menopause with fewer migraines, while others struggle with a worsening of their migraine patterns during this transition (Nappi et al., 2009).

Hormone Replacement Therapy and Migraines

Hormone replacement therapy (HRT) is sometimes used to help control menopausal symptoms, but its impact on migraines differs. Some women find relief with HRT, while others may experience more frequent migraines (Ezra & Colson, 2015).

Because there's no one-size-fits-all solution, open and honest communication with your healthcare provider is crucial. Together, you can weigh the potential benefits of HRT against any increased migraine risks or side effects you may experience. With some trial and error, patience, and a personalized approach, you can hopefully find that Goldilocks zone—the hormone balance that's just right for keeping your migraines at bay.

But if HRT ends up being more foe than friend in your migraine journey, don't be discouraged. There are so many other lifestyle strategies and treatment options to explore. The key is tuning in to the unique symphony of your body and finding what works best for you. It's all about empowering yourself with knowledge and advocating for a treatment plan that honors your personal needs and experiences.

Migraine-Stroke Risk and Vascular Health

Recent research has shed light on a concerning connection between migraines, particularly those with aura, and an increased risk of stroke and other cardiovascular events in women. Estrogen is believed to play a key role in this relationship by influencing vascular function and inflammatory pathways (Sacco et al., 2012).

Additionally, certain hormonal contraceptives containing estrogen may slightly elevate the stroke risk for some female migraineurs, particularly those who experience an aura (Champaloux et al., 2017). However, it's crucial to talk to your healthcare provider about your risks and benefits when considering contraceptive options.

Tailored Treatment Strategies

Given the profound impact hormones can have on migraines, finding the right treatment strategy is essential. Building resilience is key to raising your tolerance and reclaiming your freedom over migraines. The more you strengthen your resilience through the lifestyle strategies in this book, the better you'll be able to handle those hormonal ups and downs without ending up with a splitting migraine. This may involve a combination of acute medications for managing attacks, preventive therapies that regulate brain chemistry, and complementary approaches like supplements or mind-body techniques (Holroyd et al., 2020). Refer to Chapter 5 (stress management) and Chapter 8 (metabolic factors) for more on mind-body approaches. Similarly, you will find more information about supplements and nutrition in Chapter 7.

During major hormonal milestones like pregnancy and breastfeeding, it's vital to work closely with your doctor to ensure any migraine treatments are safe for you and your baby. Some medications may need adjusting, and exploring non-pharmacological options becomes especially important (Becker, 2018).

With professional guidance, you can develop a personalized treatment plan that accounts for your unique patterns, hormone levels, and lifestyle factors (Ripa et al., 2015). With the information provided in this book on various lifestyle approaches and mind-body techniques, you can work with your healthcare provider to incorporate complementary methods that may help address your specific needs and circumstances related to hormonal imbalances into your treatment plan.

Navigating Migraines: Holistically Steering the Hormonal Rollercoaster

For our female readers, kudos to you for taking a deep dive into the complex relationship between your hormones and migraines. I know it's not an easy road, with all the ups and downs our bodies go through from menstrual cycles to pregnancy, postpartum, and menopause. Those hormonal curveballs can either provide blissful migraine-free stretches or feel like a brutal migraine ambush.

But here's the thing—you're not powerless against these hormonally driven attacks. While you can't control Mother Nature's hormonal agenda, you can take charge of how you respond to it. It all starts with getting to know your migraine patterns like the back of your hand and building a solid partnership with your doctor.

Think of it as assembling your migraine-fighting dream team—one that's custom built to tackle your unique needs and experiences. Because let's be real, every woman's hormone saga is a little different, right?

Your Migraine Lifestyle Makeover

Now that we've mastered how hormones work, it's time to look into some lifestyle super-skills that can help you manage those hormonally triggered migraines. Think of this as your migraine lifestyle makeover:

- **Consider safe treatment options:** Complementary and alternative treatments are beneficial for women in all life stages. Pregnant women with migraines may especially benefit from non-pharmacological strategies, including meditation, and may also consider acute pain medicine or occipital nerve block for acute relief, but this option needs to be discussed with the treating doctor.

- **Become a cycle-tracking queen:** Keeping a detailed migraine diary will help you identify patterns and pinpoint any hormonal connections. When did those migraines strike compared to your cycle? What other factors played a role? This inside information is gold.

- **Namaste your stress away:** Hormones and stress are an explosive combo for migraines, so make time for serious stress-relieving practices like meditation, yoga, or just some deep belly breaths. A calmer mind is a happier mind (and body!). If you're eager to learn more, refer to the Appendix at the end of this book, which includes bonuses to help you master your meditation and breathwork practices.

- **Prioritize your beauty sleep:** Lack of sleep is like throwing fuel on the migraine fire, especially when your hormones are all over the place. Establishing good sleep habits and creating a dreamy sleep sanctuary can work wonders. Make sure that you keep to the same bedtime and wake time daily.

- **Hydrate like a queen:** Being even a little dehydrated can amplify migraines, so keep that water flowing—especially during your cycle when fluid retention can leave you feeling blah.

- **Move your body:** Regular exercise helps regulate those hormone levels and keeps migraines at bay. Find an activity you enjoy so it doesn't feel like a chore.

- **Consider Mother Nature's migraine aids:** Supplements like magnesium, riboflavin, and CoQ10 may offer some extra migraine relief—just run it by your doctor first.

- **Treat your body like a temple:** Nourishing your body with a balanced, nutrient-rich diet can stabilize your hormones and blood sugar, and can cool down inflammation. Avoid sketchy food triggers—you will score migraine brownie points.

- **Get your Zen on:** Don't underestimate the power of complementary therapies like acupuncture, massage, or mindfulness practices to help you sail through those hormonal storms.

- **Just say no to smoking (especially with HRT):** If you're a smoker using HRT, this dynamic duo could seriously increase your risk of stroke and other cardiovascular issues. The best option for your health is to stop smoking.

The key here is being open to exploring different strategies until you find your unique hormonal migraine strategy. It might take some trial and error, but that's all part of the journey to make peace with your body's hormonal rhythm.

Key Takeaways

- **Hormonal fluctuations:** Throughout different life stages like the menstrual cycle, pregnancy, postpartum period, and menopause these fluctuations can significantly impact migraine patterns and susceptibility in women.

- **Menstrual migraines:** Many women experience menstrual migraines either before or during their period, due to the dramatic drop in estrogen levels.

- **Maintaining blood sugar levels:** Hormone fluctuations during the menstrual cycle can disrupt your body's ability to regulate blood sugar levels properly, contributing to migraines. Maintaining stable blood sugar through diet and exercise may help prevent menstrual migraines.

- **Temporary migraine relief:** Pregnancy often provides relief from migraines, especially after the first trimester, likely due to sustained high estrogen levels. However, the postpartum period with rapidly plummeting hormones can trigger a resurgence of migraines.

- **Consult with your doctor about hormonally triggered migraines:** During the menopausal transition, erratic hormone fluctuations may increase the risk of hormonally triggered migraines, but the impact of hormone replacement therapy (HRT) on migraines is highly individualized and should be discussed with your doctor.

- **Increased risk of stroke and cardiovascular events:** Migraines, particularly those with aura, may be associated with an increased risk of stroke and cardiovascular events in women, potentially influenced by the role of estrogen on vascular function and inflammation.

- **Decide on a personalized, holistic treatment plan:** Working closely with a healthcare provider is crucial for developing a personalized treatment plan that accounts for hormonal changes, incorporates safe options during pregnancy/breastfeeding, and may involve a combination of acute medications, preventive therapies, and complementary approaches.

- **Implementing lifestyle strategies:** Cycle tracking, stress management, proper hydration, exercise, and a balanced diet can help women manage hormonally driven migraines and build resilience to hormonal fluctuations. For example, you may use this approach, to "dial in" with your lifestyle measures particularly during the times approaching your menstrual cycle when you may be more prone to migraines.

The interplay between migraines and hormones is complex. However, with professional guidance and a personalized treatment strategy, many women can lessen their hormonally triggered misery.

*****

In the upcoming chapter, we will explore the role of nutrition in managing your headaches. We'll talk about which foods to include in your diet and which you should rather avoid, and we will discuss how to distinguish the two categories through elimination.

Chapter 7:
Nourishing Your Way to Relief

Anything you eat or drink can either harm or help you. Certain foods or drinks may trigger your sensitivity toward migraines, while others may reduce your chances of experiencing symptoms. How will you know the difference?

Let's talk about what you should or shouldn't eat, how to identify your triggers, and what you can do to boost your nutrition to support a migraine-free life.

The Role of Nutrition in Managing Migraines

Have you ever felt unwell after eating a specific food? Did you know that migraines are triggered by food sensitivities or allergies? For some, avoiding certain foods like wheat, oranges, eggs, cheese, chocolates, and milk can help reduce the frequency, severity, and timing of migraines. Other foods, like chocolate, fatty foods, processed foods (like meat and cheese), and those with MSG can also cause migraines (Hindiyeh et al., 2020).

Taking dietary supplements and vitamins like zinc, vitamin B6, folate, magnesium, vitamin B12, vitamin C, vitamin E, and vitamin D can help prevent migraines (Crida, n.d.). The top three research-backed supplements for preventing migraines are riboflavin (vitamin B2), CoQ10, and magnesium. These help with producing energy in your body to support your brain and aids with cell activity (Gross et al., 2019).

Not everyone's migraines are triggered by the same things, and everyone's response to triggers is different. So, people with migraines need to keep track of their headaches and what they eat to figure out what might be causing their migraines and adjust their diet accordingly (Diamond & Marcus, 2016).

A balanced diet is super important for staying healthy and can help with headaches, especially for people who get migraines. Eating a mix of fruits, veggies, whole grains, lean proteins, and good fats gives your body the right tools it needs to stay healthy and might stop migraines by lowering inflammation and keeping you at a healthy weight. It's also a good idea to stay away from any foods and drinks that trigger or worsen your migraines (Hindiyeh et al., 2020; NHS, 2022).

Some diets, like ones where you cut out certain foods temporarily (elimination) or focus on high-fat, low-carb foods have shown they could help with migraines by letting you home in on what triggers them and reducing the frequency of your headaches. Also, getting enough calcium, vitamin D, and omega-3 fats in your diet can keep your teeth, bones, and heart strong, which might help with headaches, too (NHS Health Scotland, 2023).

Relieving Migraines With Essential Nutrients

Let's explore how coenzyme Q10, omega-3 fatty acids, magnesium, and vitamin B2 (riboflavin) can help you manage your migraines.

- **CoQ10:** This plays a significant role in cellular energy metabolism within the body. Current findings indicate it could be a valuable preventative measure; however, additional research is needed for further clarification. A dose of 150 mg daily is recommended to start with (The Migraine Trust, n.d.–b).

- **Omega-3 fatty acids**: These are good for reducing inflammation and can help make migraines less severe and frequent. Studies have found that omega-3 fatty acids can lower levels of certain substances in the body that cause inflammation. The doses tested in clinical trials vary (Maghsoumi-Norouzabad et al., 2017). A good starting point would be 1000 mg of omega-

3, discussed with your healthcare practitioner, if possible guided by the omega-3 index (Brown, 2022).

- **Magnesium**: This is a mineral that helps enzymes work better and plays a role in many cell activities. It's a low-cost and safe option for preventing migraines. Administering magnesium through a vein (intravenous) has been proven to help treat migraines, especially in people with low levels of magnesium in their blood (Yablon & Mauskop, 2011). The daily dose of magnesium for migraines is recommended at 600 mg (The Migraine Trust, n.d.–b). I have also written a book on magnesium. If you are interested in diving deeper into its benefits, see the Appendix at the end of this book.

- **Vitamin B2:** This supplement, also known as riboflavin, is crucial for producing energy in our cells and could help prevent migraines. It's safe for most people and might lower the intensity and reoccurrence of migraines for some individuals. The NICE Clinical Guidelines suggest taking 400 mg of riboflavin daily to prevent migraines (NICE, n.d.).

Even though these nutrients can help with migraines by reducing inflammation, you also need to do your part by maintaining a healthy weight and avoiding the specific foods that can trigger them. Remember, before trying any new supplements, it's important to consult with your doctor to ensure they are safe and effective for you.

Dietary Approaches and Meal Planning for Migraine Relief

Adopting a dietary approach tailored to migraine management can be a powerful tool in your journey toward relief. By exploring various eating patterns and incorporating migraine-friendly foods and nutrients, you can potentially reduce inflammation, regulate brain chemistry, and minimize the frequency and severity of your migraine episodes.

- **Low-Inflammatory diets:** Chronic inflammation has been linked to various health issues, including migraines. By adopting a low-inflammatory diet, you can reduce your consumption of foods that contribute to inflammation and prioritize anti-inflammatory options.

- **Plant-based diets:** These diets have gained popularity for their role in reducing inflammation, and promoting overall wellness. These diets are rich in antioxidants, fiber, and phytochemicals, which may help regulate brain function and reduce migraine triggers.

- **Mediterranean diet:** The Mediterranean diet, renowned for its heart-healthy benefits, has also shown promise in migraine management.

We have covered a few dietary approaches here to get you started. For those of you interested in learning more about how diet and nutrition may help prevent or reduce migraine headaches, an insightful research paper on this topic was published in 2022. Titled "Migraine Headaches: Opportunities for Management With Precision Nutrition" by Dr. Benjamin Brown in the NUTRITION MEDICINE JOURNAL, this comprehensive review explores dietary strategies and methods of personalized nutrition that show promise for migraine treatment.

Because everyone's diet is unique, it's important for each person to take a personalized approach and pay attention to how they feel. Focus on eating whole foods, including a variety of colorful plants, while cutting down on sugar and processed foods. In Chapter 8, we will talk some more about why it's so important to stabilize your blood sugar with regular meals and snacks. For now, let's explore some practical examples of the above-mentioned dietary approaches that will help you do this.

Healthier Eating Strategies

The Mediterranean, DASH, and MIND diets are two dietary patterns that have been associated with potential benefits for brain health and migraine prevention.

Mediterranean Diet

The Mediterranean diet is influenced by the long-standing dietary practices of individuals residing in nations that surround the Mediterranean Sea. It emphasizes:

- plant-based foods like fruits, vegetables, whole grains, legumes, nuts, and seeds.

- using olive oil as the main source of healthy fats.

- moderate amounts of fish, poultry, dairy, and red wine.

- limited intake of red meat, sweets, and processed foods.

The Mediterranean diet is rich in antioxidants, fiber, healthy fats, and anti-inflammatory compounds that may help regulate metabolic pathways linked to migraines.

DASH Diet

The Dietary Approaches to Stop Hypertension (DASH) diet was initially created to aid in the treatment and prevention of high blood pressure (hypertension). It has also been associated with other potential health benefits, including reduced risk of certain chronic diseases and migraine prevention.

The DASH diet focuses on:

- vegetables and fruits

- whole grains

- low-fat dairy

- lean meats, fish, poultry

- nuts, seeds, and legumes

- limited amounts of fats, red meats, sweets, and sodium

Specifically, the DASH diet recommends consuming daily, up to (The Nutrition Source, n.d.):

- five portions of fruits

- five portions of vegetables

- eight portions of whole grains

- three servings of low-fat dairy, and

- limited sodium (2,300 mg per day or lower)

By focusing on nutrient-rich foods that are high in fiber, minerals like magnesium and potassium, and beneficial fats, the DASH diet helps reduce inflammation and oxidative stress in the body. This anti-inflammatory effect is thought to be one of the mechanisms by which it may help prevent migraines.

Additionally, the DASH diet promotes healthy blood pressure levels and improved vascular function, which could also play a role in migraine pathophysiology related to blood vessel changes.

Overall, like the Mediterranean diet, the DASH diet's emphasis on wholesome, plant-forward eating may help regulate metabolic processes and maintain the balanced neurochemistry needed to reduce migraine episodes.

MIND Diet

The Mediterranean-DASH Intervention for Neurodegenerative Delay (MIND) diet is a hybrid of the Mediterranean and DASH diets, designed to promote brain health.

It recommends eating:

- green leafy vegetables and other veggies, nuts, berries, beans, whole grains, olive oil, fish, and poultry (if you prefer to include meat)

And limits intake of:

- red meats, butter and margarine, cheese, sweets and other sugary food, and fried or fast foods

By combining aspects of the Mediterranean and DASH diets, the MIND diet aims to reduce oxidative stress, inflammation, and cardiovascular risk factors (Pearson & Burford, 2023)—all of which may play a role in migraine pathogenesis.

These diets emphasize nutrient-dense plant foods, healthy fats, and lean proteins while limiting processed, sugary, and fried items. Their anti-inflammatory and neuroprotective effects may help optimize metabolic function and reduce migraine frequency and severity for some individuals.

Supplementation

But diet is just one piece of the puzzle. Have you looked into migraine-busting supplements? Powerhouse nutrients like co-enzyme Q10 (CoQ10), riboflavin, and magnesium could bolster mitochondrial function, slash oxidative stress, and promote better insulin sensitivity—hitting those metabolic keys associated with migraines. The above section covered these and their doses in detail. First, discuss with your doctor before hopping on any new supplement routines.

Migraine-Friendly Meal Planning

One of the best ways to incorporate migraine-friendly foods and nutrients into your daily routine is through delicious and nutritious smoothies, meals, and snacks. Here are some ideas to help you nourish your way to migraine relief by building your meal plans.

On-the-Go Smoothie Recipes

Adding fruit and greens with seeds and other wholesome ingredients can help you consume what your body needs through easy-as-pie smoothies.

Berry-Licious Blend

For a refreshing and nutrient-packed beverage, combine the following ingredients in your powerful blender:

- 1/2 cup of plain yogurt

- 1 cup of berries (any variety)

- 1 cup of almond milk (unsweetened)

- A handful of spinach

- 1 tbsp of chia seeds

- 1 tsp of honey for a touch of sweetness (if desired)

Blend these components until they form a well-incorporated, velvety consistency, and enjoy.

Tropical Kale Bliss

- 1 cup of coconut milk (unsweetened)

- 1/2 cup of plain yogurt

- 1 cup of mango chunks

- 1/2 tsp of ground ginger

- A handful of kale

- 1 tbsp of chia seeds

Beat it all in your high-speed blender and enjoy.

Breakfast Recipes

Let's explore some nutrient-dense and migraine-friendly breakfast options.

Overnight Oats with Mixed Berries and Chia Seeds

The evening before:

- 1 cup of rolled oats (gluten-free if you are sensitive to it)

- 1/2 cup of almond milk

- 1/2 cup of yogurt

- 1 tsp of chia seeds

- 1 tsp of vanilla extract

The next morning:

- 1/2 cup of fresh berries

- 1 tsp of honey (optional)

- 1 tsp of nuts (optional)

Instructions

1. Add the ingredients for the evening-before in a glass jar or lidded bowl, and blend properly.

2. Cover the jar or bowl and refrigerate overnight (or for at least four to six hours).

3. In the morning, give the overnight oats a good stir to incorporate any liquid that may have separated.

4. Add fresh mixed berries to the oats.

5. If you're seeking an extra touch of sweetness, consider drizzling some honey (at most one tablespoon) over it.

6. Top with sliced almonds or other nuts of your choice for an extra crunch.

7. Enjoy your delicious and nutritious overnight oats!

Notes

- Adjust your amount of milk or yogurt to achieve the desired consistency.

- You can experiment with different types of berries or fruits subject to what you like and seasonal availability.

- For added fiber and omega-3s, consider mixing in a tablespoon of ground flaxseed or chia seeds.

This overnight oats recipe is not only migraine-friendly but also packed with nutrients from whole grains, berries, and chia seeds. The combination of complex carbohydrates, fiber, and healthy fats can help control blood sugar levels and provide ongoing energy throughout the morning.

Spinach and Mushroom Frittata with Whole-Grain Toast

The combination of eggs, vegetables, and whole grains provides a balanced mix of protein, fiber, and complex carbohydrates, making it a satisfying and nourishing start to your day.

Ingredients

- 1/4 cup of milk or plant-based alternative, unsweetened
- 1/2 tsp of salt
- 1/4 tsp of ground black pepper
- 1 tbsp of olive oil
- 5 extra-large eggs
- 1 cup of mushrooms, sliced
- 1 clove of garlic, minced
- 2 cups of baby spinach
- crumbled feta cheese (optional)
- whole-grain bread slices (toasted)

Instructions

Preheat your oven to 375 °F (190 °C).

1. Using a bowl, whisk together the unsweetened milk/alternative, eggs, ground black pepper, and salt until they form a cohesive and well-incorporated mixture. Set aside.

2. Heat the olive oil in a 9-inch oven-safe skillet or baking dish over medium heat.

3. Toss the sliced mushrooms and minced garlic into the skillet. Let them cook for around 4 minutes.

4. Throw in the fresh baby spinach leaves and keep cooking for about 3 more minutes until the spinach gets all wilted and soft.

5. Pour that eggy mixture right over the top of the sauteed veggies, spreading it out evenly across the skillet.

6. Jazz it up with crumbled feta on top of the frittata, if desired.

7. Once you've got everything in the skillet, slide it into the oven that you preheated earlier. Let it bake for 15 to 20 minutes, until the frittata looks set and a little puffed up.

8. Take the frittata out of the oven. Let it cool for a few minutes. While it's cooling, toast the whole-grain bread.

9. Cut the frittata into wedges and dish up warm, alongside the toast.

Notes

- Substitute with other vegetables, such as bell peppers, onions, or tomatoes.

- For a dairy-free option, omit the feta cheese or use a vegan cheese alternative.

- Whole-grain bread provides complex carbohydrates and fiber, which can help regulate blood sugar levels and support migraine management.

Low-Inflammatory Lunch Recipes

Lentil and Sweet Potato Soup With a Side of Mixed Greens

This soup with mixed greens is a satisfying and nutrient-dense meal that is both migraine-friendly and packed with plant-based goodness. The combination of lentils, sweet potatoes, and a variety of vegetables provides a range of vitamins, minerals, and fiber, while the mixed greens salad adds a fresh and crisp element to the dish.

Ingredients

- 1 onion, diced
- 2 small sweet potatoes, peeled and chopped
- 3 cloves of garlic, minced
- 1 cup of lentils, dried and rinsed
- 3-4 carrots, peeled and sliced into discs
- 2 celery stalks, sliced
- 1 tsp of ground cumin
- 1/2 tsp of smoked paprika
- 4 cups of vegetable or chicken broth
- 2 cups of water
- salt and black pepper, to taste
- 2 cups of mixed greens
- 2 red bell peppers, diced
- 1 tbsp of balsamic vinegar
- 1 tbsp of olive oil

Instructions

1. In a large pot, combine the lentils, diced sweet potato, onion, garlic, carrots, celery, cumin, smoked paprika, broth, and water.

2. Cook over high heat until boiling, then reduce the heat to low, cover your pot, and let it simmer for about 20 to 25 minutes, or until the lentils and vegetables are tender.

3. Once the lentils and vegetables are cooked, use an immersion blender or transfer a portion of the soup to a blender and purée until you reach your desired consistency. (Alternatively, you can leave the soup as is for a heartier texture.)

4. Flavor your soup with black pepper and salt, to taste.

5. In a separate bowl, combine the mixed greens, red bell peppers, olive oil, and balsamic vinegar. Toss the dressing over the greens.

6. Serve the lentil and sweet potato soup hot, accompanied by the mixed greens salad on the side.

Notes

- For a creamier texture, stir in a dollop of plain Greek yogurt or a splash of unsweetened plant-based milk.

- If you prefer a spicier soup, you can add chili flakes or some cayenne pepper, too.

- The mixed greens salad provides a refreshing contrast to the warm soup and adds additional nutrients and fiber to the meal.

- Replace the greens with a side of whole-grain bread or crackers if you like.

Quinoa Salad and Grilled Salmon

This salad with grilled salmon is a nutritious and migraine-friendly meal that combines lean protein from the salmon with the fiber-rich and nutrient-dense quinoa salad.

Ingredients

- 2 cups of veggie broth or water

- 1 cup of tomatoes, halved

- 1 cup of cucumber, diced

- 1/2 cup of onion, diced

- 1/4 cup of fresh parsley, chopped

- 1 tsp of Dijon mustard

- 2 tbsp of lime juice

- 2 tbsp of avocado oil

- 1 cup of quinoa, rinsed

- salt and pepper

For the salmon:

- 2 tbsp of avocado oil

- 4 salmon fillets

- 1 tsp of dried dill

- salt and pepper

Instructions

1. Preheat your grill or oven to 400 °F.

2. Prepare the salmon: Brush the fillets with olive oil and sprinkle with salt, dried dill, and pepper.

3. In the preheated oven, grill the salmon fillets for a maximum of 15 minutes (or bake for a maximum of 18 minutes) until they are cooked through and flaky.

4. In the meantime, cook the quinoa. In a saucepan, combine the quinoa and water or vegetable broth.

5. Lower the heat once it's come to a boil, cover, and simmer for about 15 minutes, or until the quinoa is fluffy and all the liquid absorbed.

6. Separate grains with a fork and place them in a bowl to cool down.

7. Prepare your lemon vinaigrette: In a bowl, whip together the Dijon mustard, lime juice, olive oil, salt, and pepper.

8. Assemble the quinoa salad: Add the cherry tomatoes, cucumber, red onion, and chopped parsley to the slightly cooled quinoa.

9. Drizzle with the lime vinaigrette and toss gently to combine. Serve the grilled salmon with the salad.

Notes

- For extra flavor, marinate the salmon in a mixture of olive oil, lemon juice, garlic, and herbs before grilling or baking.

- Feel free to add other vegetables to the quinoa salad, such as bell peppers, avocado, or roasted vegetables.

- If you prefer a warmer salad, you can add the vinaigrette to the quinoa while it's still warm, and toss in the remaining ingredients.

Nutritional Snack Options

- Make skewers with fresh fruit and serve with yogurt as a sauce

- Enjoy cucumber with hummus

- Dip carrot sticks in guacamole

- Mix up some unsalted nuts, seeds, and dried fruit, and grab a handful for a quick energy boost.

Migraine-Friendly Dinner Dishes

Ginger Chickpea Stir-Fry

A decent choice for a migraine-friendly dinner is the ginger chickpea stir-fry. This dish incorporates sautéed chickpeas mixed with fresh ginger, garlic, and assorted vegetables. By sautéing these ingredients together, you enhance the flavors and create a nutritious meal that is gentle on migraine triggers. The presence of ginger in this dish not only adds a zesty taste but also offers potential benefits for migraine relief due to its anti-inflammatory properties.

Instructions

- **Sauté chickpeas:** Start by heating a pan with a bit of oil and adding the chickpeas until they turn slightly brown and crisp.

- **Add flavors:** Incorporate the fresh ginger and garlic into the pan, allowing their aromas to infuse with the chickpeas.

- **Mix in vegetables:** Add a variety of colorful vegetables such as bell peppers, broccoli, and carrots for added texture and nutrients.

- **Serve over grains:** To make it a complete meal, serve the ginger chickpea stir-fry over a bed of brown rice or quinoa.

This adds a satisfying base to your dish and ensures a balanced intake of carbohydrates and proteins.

Baked Cod with Roasted Vegetables

Ingredients

For the Baked Cod

- 4 cod fillets
- 3 cloves of garlic, minced
- 1 lemon, sliced
- Fresh herbs, chopped
- Salt and pepper to taste
- Olive oil

For the Roasted Vegetables

- 2 large sweet potatoes, peeled and diced
- 1 lb Brussels sprouts, trimmed and halved
- 4 large carrots, peeled and sliced
- Olive oil
- Salt and pepper to taste
- 1 tbsp honey
- Fresh thyme or rosemary

Instructions

Baking the cod:

Preheat the oven to 400 °F (200 °C).

1. Place the cod fillets on a baking sheet lined with parchment paper.

2. Drizzle the cod with olive oil and season with minced garlic, salt, and pepper.

3. Lay lemon slices and sprinkle fresh herbs over the cod fillets.

4. Bake in the preheated oven for 15-20 minutes, or until the fish is tender and flakes easily with a fork.

Roasting the sweet potatoes:

Preheat the oven to 400 °F (200 °C) if not already done.

1. In a bowl, toss the diced sweet potatoes with olive oil, salt, and pepper.

2. Spread the sweet potato cubes in a single layer on a baking sheet.

3. Roast for 25-30 minutes, or until crispy on the outside and tender inside, turning halfway through.

Roasting the Brussels sprouts:

Preheat the oven to 400 °F (200 °C) if not already done.

1. Toss the halved Brussels sprouts with olive oil, salt, and pepper.

2. Arrange them cut side down on a baking sheet. Roast for 20 to 25 minutes, or until crispy and caramelized, shaking the pan halfway through.

Roasting the carrots:

Preheat the oven to 400 °F (200 °C) if not already done.

1. Toss the sliced carrots with olive oil, honey, and a sprinkle of thyme or rosemary. Spread the carrots on a baking sheet.

2. Roast for 20 to 25 minutes, or until tender and caramelized, turning halfway through. Plate the baked cod fillets alongside the roasted sweet potatoes, Brussels sprouts, and carrots.

3. Garnish with a sprinkle of fresh herbs or a drizzle of lemon juice for added brightness. Serve and enjoy this wholesome and flavorful meal with your family and friends.

Tips for Meal Planning

-   Plan your meals and snacks to ensure a consistent and balanced intake of nutrients.

-   Incorporate a variety of migraine-friendly foods from different food groups.

-   Prioritize foods rich in omega-3 fatty acids, magnesium, riboflavin, and other migraine-relieving nutrients.

-   Keep your body well hydrated by sipping on water throughout the day. Opt for nature's refreshment instead of sugary beverages like sodas or fruit juices that can contribute to an undesirable spike in your blood sugar levels.

-   Monitor your food intake and adjust your meal plan as needed based on your migraine triggers and responses.

-   Drink a tea that helps fight inflammation, like green tea or ginger tea.

- Make sure to eat regularly and don't miss meals, specifically if you have noticed that this induces or worsens your migraines.

- Consider eating five reduced-portion-size meals per day.

- Eat a carbohydrate with a protein or a good fat to stay full longer.

Identifying Dietary Triggers: A Personal Journey

As great as the right foods can be for managing your migraines, the wrong foods may cause detrimental health effects, making your migraine events even worse.

Uncovering the foods or ingredients that may contribute to your migraine episodes can be a game-changer in managing your condition. While the process requires patience and diligence, the rewards can be invaluable—a better understanding of your unique triggers and the ability to make informed choices to reduce the frequency and severity of your migraines.

Keeping a Food Diary: Your Personal Migraine Detective

Remember how we discussed that keeping a journal is an important tool in migraine management? Imagine having a trusty notebook by your side, ready to document every morsel that passes your lips and every migraine episode that rears its unwelcome head. This food diary becomes your migraine detective, helping you spot patterns and correlations between what you consume and the onset of those debilitating headaches.

Here are some tips to make the most of your food diary:

- **Be diligent and consistent:** Jot down your meals and snacks immediately after eating, and document migraine symptoms as soon as they strike. Accuracy is key.

- **Include portion sizes:** Note the approximate amounts of each food or beverage to help identify potential trigger quantities.

- **Provide details:** Don't just list the main ingredients—include condiments, seasonings, and any additives used in the preparation.

- **Note other factors:** Record your stress levels, sleep patterns, and environmental factors, as these may also contribute to migraine episodes.

By consistently tracking your food intake and migraine occurrences, you may shed light on your personal triggers.

The Elimination Diet: Following a Targeted Approach

If you suspect certain foods or food groups may be behind your migraines, an elimination diet or food challenge can provide more definitive answers. This approach involves removing potential trigger foods from your diet for a set period and then reintroducing them one by one, carefully observing any reactions.

Here's how you should do it:

- **Identify potential trigger foods:** Based on your food diary or existing knowledge, create a list of foods or food groups you suspect may be triggers.

- **Eliminate trigger foods:** Remove the identified foods from your diet for a specified period, typically two to four weeks.

- **Reintroduce foods one by one:** After the elimination period, reintroduce the removed foods one at a time, allowing several days between each reintroduction to monitor for any migraine symptoms or reactions.

- **Observe and document:** Carefully track any migraine episodes or adverse reactions that occur after reintroducing each food.

- **Repeat as you need to:** If no reactions occur, move on to the next suspected trigger food. If a reaction is observed, eliminate that food from your diet and consider further testing, if needed.

It's important to note that elimination diets and food challenges should be undertaken with the guidance of a healthcare professional or registered dietitian, as they can be complex and may require adjustments to ensure proper nutrient intake.

Common Culprits: Foods to Watch Out For

While dietary triggers can be unique to each person, certain foods and ingredients have been identified as common migraine triggers. Some culprits include aged cheeses, processed meats, artificial sweeteners, MSG, and alcohol.

Remember, identifying your dietary triggers is a journey of self-discovery. By diligently tracking your food intake and migraine episodes, and by working closely with a healthcare professional or registered dietitian, you can uncover the foods or ingredients that may be contributing to your migraines and make informed adjustments to your diet for better overall management of your condition.

Hydration and Migraines: Quenching Your Thirst for Relief

When it comes to managing migraines, the importance of proper hydration cannot be overstated. Our bodies are composed of approximately 60% water, and even mild dehydration can have far-reaching effects, including the potential to trigger or exacerbate migraine episodes.

The Hydration-Migraine Connection

Dehydration can be a significant contributing factor to migraine headaches. When our bodies don't receive enough fluids, the delicate balance of electrolytes and other essential compounds can be disrupted, leading to changes in brain chemistry and function. These imbalances can potentially trigger a cascade of events that culminate in the onset of a migraine attack.

Moreover, dehydration can cause the brain to shrink slightly, pulling away from the skull and creating irritation and inflammation of the surrounding membranes and nerves. This physical stress on the brain and its protective layers can further exacerbate migraine symptoms.

Staying Hydrated: A Simple Yet Powerful Solution

The solution to mitigating the effects of dehydration on migraines is relatively simple: Consume plenty of water and maintain optimal hydration levels throughout the day. By maintaining adequate fluid intake, you can help regulate brain chemistry, prevent electrolyte imbalances, and reduce the physical stress on your brain and its surrounding structures.

Here are some strategies to help you stay hydrated and potentially reduce the frequency and severity of your migraine episodes:

- **Bring your water bottle everywhere:** Keep a reusable water bottle close at all times, and make a conscious effort to drink from it regularly throughout the day.

- **Create reminders:** Use your phone or smartwatch to set reminders to drink water regularly, ensuring consistent hydration.

- **Eat hydrating foods:** Incorporate water-rich fruits and vegetables, such as watermelon, cucumber, and berries, into your diet to contribute to your overall fluid intake.

- **Monitor urine color:** Pay attention to the color of your urine— pale yellow or nearly clear urine is an indication of adequate hydration, while darker shades may signal dehydration.

- **Consider electrolyte drinks:** In addition to water, consider incorporating beverages rich in electrolytes like aloe vera or coconut water, especially during periods of increased perspiration or physical activity.

While staying hydrated is crucial for migraine management, it's essential to consult with your healthcare provider or a registered dietitian to ensure you're meeting your individual hydration needs and addressing any underlying medical conditions that may contribute to dehydration or migraine episodes.

When you make hydration a priority and incorporate strategies to increase your fluid intake, you can take an important step toward managing your migraines and improving your overall well-being.

Support for Dietary Approaches and Nutrition

Let's explore some practical tools and resources for managing migraines through dietary approaches and nutrition. Keep an eye out for the Bonus chapter where we will be discussing more practical tools and resources.

- **Meal planning apps:** Use apps like Mealime or Plan to Eat to create meal plans that align with anti-inflammatory, nutrient-dense diets. These apps can help you incorporate migraine-friendly foods into your diet while avoiding common triggers.

- **Food tracking apps:** Apps like MyFitnessPal or Migraine Buddy can help you track your food intake and migraine symptoms. This can help you more effectively recognize the patterns and potential triggers that precede your migraines.

- **Online communities and forums:** Join online communities or forums dedicated to migraine management and dietary approaches. These platforms can provide support, tips, and recipes from others who have had similar experiences.

- **Cookbooks and recipe websites:** Look for cookbooks and websites that focus on migraine-friendly recipes. These resources can help you prepare delicious meals that align with your dietary goals. See the Appendix for information about my upcoming migraine cookbook.

- **Nutritional counseling:** Consult with a registered dietitian who practices in the field of migraine management and treatment. They can provide personalized guidance and support to help you optimize your diet for migraine prevention.

- **Hydration tracking apps:** Use apps like WaterMinder or Hydro Coach to track your daily water intake. These apps can help you stay hydrated, which is important for migraine prevention.

By leveraging these tools and resources, you can effectively incorporate dietary strategies into your migraine management plan and improve your overall quality of life.

Key Takeaways

- **Healthy eating:** Eating a balanced diet rich in nutrients can help reduce the frequency and intensity of migraines. The Mediterranean or MIND diets, which focus on whole foods like fruits, vegetables, and whole grains, may be particularly beneficial.

- **Food diary:** Keeping track of what you eat and when you get migraines can help you identify and avoid potential triggers.

- **Stay hydrated:** Drinking enough water throughout the day can help prevent migraines triggered by dehydration.

- **Consider supplements:** Some supplements like magnesium, riboflavin (vitamin B2), and CoQ10 may help with migraine management, but it's important to talk to your healthcare provider before starting any new supplement regimen.

- **Get professional advice:** Consulting with a registered dietitian or healthcare provider can help you create a personalized diet plan that supports your migraine management goals.

- **Personalized approach:** What works for one person may not work for another, so it's important to listen to your body and find the approach that works best for you.

By making these adjustments to your lifestyle and diet, you can nourish your body in a way that supports migraine management and improves your overall well-being.

*****

In our next chapter, we're shifting gears to explore another fascinating piece of the migraine puzzle—the role of metabolic factors. We'll dive into how underlying conditions like metabolic disorders, biochemical imbalances, and nutritional deficiencies could be potential migraine culprits.

Understanding the metabolic influences can give you a better idea of what might trigger your migraines. And guess what? It means you'll have more strategies to fight them! So get ready, because this journey into metabolism is just beginning.

Chapter 8:
Metabolic Factors Contributing to Migraines

Ever wonder why certain foods or habits have the ability to trigger headaches? Our body's metabolic processes hold the answer. From blood sugar swings to hormonal imbalances, internal factors work with these elements to bring about migraines.

Metabolism contributes to migraines, beyond genetics and classic triggers. Conditions like insulin resistance and obesity are linked to migraine susceptibility. Metabolic syndrome, with obesity and cholesterol imbalances, can influence migraine development. Mitochondrial dysfunction and metabolic disruptions may also impact migraine episodes.

In this chapter, we delve into these metabolic factors contributing to headaches, peeling back the layers to better understand their impact. We'll explore how blood sugar stability, hormone cycles, hydration, and other elements can either mitigate or exacerbate migraines. By the end of this chapter, you'll have a clearer picture of how your body's internal processes relate to those debilitating headaches and what steps you can take to manage them more effectively. And for those looking to dive even deeper, see the appendix for a couple of relevant books in my Brain Health series.

The Metabolic Roots of Migraines

As we continue unraveling migraine's complexities, shining a light on these often-overlooked metabolic influences may be a game-changer. It could pave the way for new therapies and a deeper grasp of what drives this multifaceted neurological condition that impacts so many lives. Let's find out more about the above, and what these complex terms mean.

Glucose Metabolism

Let's discuss glucose metabolism. Glucose is the main fuel that keeps our bodies running. When your blood sugar levels drop too low, a condition known as hypoglycemia, your brain may not get the energy it requires to function optimally. This can lead to symptoms like dizziness, confusion, and yes, even headaches.

Conversely, high blood sugar levels can also trigger headaches due to fluctuations that stress your body's metabolism. A balanced diet that maintains stable blood sugar levels is crucial. Consider snacks that combine protein, healthy fats, and complex carbohydrates to keep your glucose steady throughout the day.

Insulin Resistance and Obesity

Insulin resistance refers to a condition where the body's cells become resistant to the effects of insulin, a hormone that regulates blood sugar levels. As a result, higher levels of insulin are needed to metabolize glucose effectively. Insulin resistance is connected to obesity, type 2 diabetes, and metabolic syndrome.

Insulin resistance and obesity seem to increase your risk of suffering more frequent migraines and other headache types. When your body becomes resistant to insulin's effects in regulating blood sugar levels, it can set off a metabolic domino effect. Your blood sugar ends up on a roller coaster of highs and lows, while your body enters a state of chronic inflammation as it tries to compensate.

This inflammatory, high-sugar environment takes a toll. It creates high levels of oxidative stress that can harm cells and proteins. It impairs the healthy function of blood vessels, making it harder for them to dilate and constrict properly. And it disrupts the delicate neurochemical balance in the brain that modulates pain pathways.

When insulin can't do its job managing blood sugar effectively, it creates physiological conditions that make your neurons more excitable, your blood vessels more unstable, and your whole system primed for inflammatory reactions—the perfect storm for triggering a migraine episode. Restoring metabolic harmony by improving insulin sensitivity may help defuse this chain reaction.

Mitochondrial Dysfunction

Now, onto mitochondrial dysfunction. Your mitochondria are the powerhouses of your cells, responsible for producing ATP, the cell's energy currency. Inefficiencies in this process can result in less energy being available to your brain, which can contribute to migraine symptoms.

With dysfunctional mitochondria, cells don't get the energizing fuel they need, leaving them depleted and struggling to work optimally. At the same time, these faulty mitochondria start spewing out harmful oxidative byproducts that can damage proteins, genes, and cellular structures. Your body's natural inflammatory response also gets kicked into overdrive trying to combat the disruption.

Researchers have found that people with mitochondrial abnormalities often have migraines, making the case for efficient cellular energy production playing a vital role in headache prevention (Wang et al., 2023). When neurons in the brain are starved of proper energy and swimming in oxidative stress, they are more excitable and prone to firing painful signals. Restoring proper mitochondrial health could help stabilize both neuronal firing and blood flow regulation.

Lipid Abnormalities

Having an out-of-whack cholesterol profile seems to put people at higher risk of frequent migraine misery. We're talking about high levels of those unhealthy triglycerides combined with suppressed levels of the "good" HDL cholesterol. This dyslipidemia, as doctors call it, can gum up the metabolic works in ways that may trigger migraines.

For one, it promotes inflammation throughout the body. And we know inflammation plays a pivotal role in activating the trigeminovascular system and pain pathways underlying migraines. This cholesterol imbalance also disrupts the normal functioning of the endothelial cells lining our blood vessels. With endothelial dysfunction, vessels can't dilate and constrict properly—another vascular component of migraines.

Dyslipidemia also alters how energy is utilized and metabolized within the brain itself. This potential energy deficiency state may make neurons more excitable and unstable.

So whether it's igniting inflammatory fires, impairing vascular flexibility, or short-circuiting proper brain energy usage, getting your cholesterol out of unhealthy ranges emerges as a potential way to restore metabolic order and help keep your migraines at bay.

Obesity and Adipokine Imbalances

Carrying extra pounds doesn't just strain your joints and organs—it may also amplify your risk of battling chronic migraines and overusing pain meds. The culprit? Those uber-active fat cells you're carrying.

Fat tissue isn't merely a passive storage space for extra calories. It's a biochemical factory pumping out inflammatory molecules called adipokines. When you've got a surplus of fat cells from obesity, those adipokine levels get skewed out of their normal balanced ranges. Visceral fat (the abdominal fat cells that surround the internal organs) is particularly harmful.

This adipokine imbalance can throw your whole metabolic system out of whack. It fuels widespread inflammation and disrupts the body's ability to maintain stable internal environments for optimal functioning.

That's a recipe for neurogenic inflammation—the excessive firing of pain neurons implicated in headache disorders like migraines.

Having excessive adipose tissue from obesity creates a constant low-grade fire of inflammation throughout your system. Those inflamed pain pathways are essentially stuck in the "on" position, making your brain hypersensitive and primed for migraine attacks.

Getting a handle on obesity may help restore proper adipokine equilibrium and metabolic homeostasis. This could help "douse" those overactive pain signals and stop the vicious cycle of chronic headaches and medication overuse. A little weight loss may go a long way in dialing down migraine misery.

Managing Magnesium Levels

As I've briefly mentioned in the previous chapters, managing your magnesium levels is another key aspect. Magnesium is a critical mineral involved in numerous biochemical reactions and metabolism in the body, including nervous system regulation. Studies have shown that individuals with low magnesium levels are more susceptible to experiencing migraines. Foods rich in magnesium like leafy greens, nuts, seeds, and whole grains can help mitigate this risk. Regularly incorporating these foods into your diet can maintain optimal mineral balance, potentially minimizing the frequency of headaches. Find out more about how to approach this in my book about magnesium. Visit the Appendix at the end of this book for more information.

The Effects of Dehydration

Let's not forget about what we've discussed about hydration in the previous chapter. Dehydration, a known headache trigger, reduces blood volume, leading to decreased blood flow and oxygen to the brain. This can cause tissues to shrink slightly, pulling away from the bone and causing pain. Drinking sufficient water daily is a simple yet effective way to prevent dehydration-induced headaches.

Electrolyte Balance

Closely related to hydration is electrolyte balance. Electrolytes like sodium, potassium, and calcium are vital for proper nerve and muscle function. An imbalance, whether from excessive sweating, poor nutrition, or other factors, can lead to headaches. Simple dietary tweaks can make a world of difference. Including electrolyte-rich foods such as bananas, avocados, and yogurt, and considering electrolyte supplements if necessary, can support overall metabolic health. Refer back to Chapter 7 for our discussion on hydration and supplementation.

Your Gut-Brain Axis

Another piece of the migraine metabolic puzzle is the gut-brain axis. The gut has its unique nervous system, the enteric nervous system, which communicates directly with the brain. Imbalances in gut bacteria can influence this communication, potentially leading to inflammation and headaches. Consuming probiotics through foods like yogurt, kefir, and fermented vegetables can improve gut health and, by extension, reduce headache occurrences. Probiotic supplements can also be beneficial; however, consult with a healthcare provider to determine what's best for you. Refer to Chapter 4 where we discussed this in more detail.

Hormone Fluctuations

The exact mechanisms linking these metabolic perturbations to migraines are still being elucidated. However, the converging effects on processes like oxidative stress, inflammation, impaired energy metabolism, and neurovascular dysfunction appear to play a crucial role in headache pathophysiology. Targeting these metabolic roots through lifestyle, dietary, and therapeutic interventions may offer new avenues for headache prevention and management. In Chapter 6, we did a comprehensive exploration of female hormones and migraines.

Stress and Sleep

Lastly, let's talk about stress and sleep. Both significantly affect metabolic processes and, subsequently, headache potential. Chronic stress can elevate cortisol levels, leading to metabolic imbalances that intensify headache frequency and severity. Sleep deprivation disrupts metabolism and places additional strain on your body, making you more prone to headaches. Prioritizing relaxation techniques like deep breathing and ensuring adequate, quality sleep each night are effective strategies for maintaining metabolic balance. You will remember we spoke about sleep in Chapter 2, and covered stress management in Chapter 5 (refer back for some helpful tips).

To wrap up, integrating natural solutions backed by evidence from holistic health can be a game-changer in managing your headaches. By taking these steps, you create a supportive environment for your body's complex systems, reducing the likelihood of headaches and enhancing overall well-being.

Holistic Methods to Treat Your Migraines

Let's be real—managing the metabolic factors behind migraines goes way beyond just taking pills. While medications have their place, a more holistic, integrative approach that embraces natural, evidence-based solutions can be a real game-changer.

Exploring complementary therapies outside of mainstream medicine can be a total game-changer. Getting creative with alternative treatments like massage, meditation, and yoga—you name it—may lead to better sleep, mood enhancement, and improved roots of metabolic factors for migraines. Some people have even been able to ditch the meds entirely by finding the right blend of natural, holistic approaches.

Of course, others combine the best of both worlds—using complementary therapies as a supportive sidekick to their prescription regimen. That one-two punch can help maximize relief.

Think about it this way: The very foods we put into our bodies influence those metabolic pathways that can trigger migraine storms when out of whack. Cleaning up your diet by loading up on brain-boosting fruits, veggies, whole grains, and healthy fats can help restore metabolic harmony. Eating strategies like the Mediterranean or MIND diets (discussed in Chapter 7) have shown serious promise in dialing down migraine intensity and frequency, likely because they prioritize anti-inflammatory, nutrient-dense fare.

Balancing Your Blood Sugar

Yes, balancing your blood sugar levels is part of the umbrella of holistic tools you can use to build your brain resilience. Let me highlight why evening out your blood sugar levels is so impactful for migraine relief.

Many of my patients and the participants in my migraine mentorship program found this approach beneficial. High blood sugar spikes followed by a rapid drop can initiate migraines. People don't often realize the connection until they look closely at the timing of their headaches plus their dietary patterns. In some cases, doctors may recommend using a continuous glucose monitor to confirm if blood sugar dysregulation is an issue.

Here are some tips to stabilize your blood sugar:

- **Start meals with vegetables:** Having veggies first slows down the absorption of carbohydrates, stabilizing blood sugar rise. Plus, dark leafy greens provide migraine-relieving magnesium.

- **Smart snacking:** Options like an apple with nut butter or berries and nuts can keep blood sugar levels steady between meals.

- **Post-meal walks:** After a carb-rich meal, gentle movement like a walk helps to stabilize your blood sugar levels.

- **Healthy fats:** Include sources like fatty fish, nuts, seeds, avocado, and olive oil. The healthy fats and omega-3s nourish the brain while moderating blood sugar impacts.

Balancing and stabilizing blood sugar through these dietary and lifestyle adjustments can substantially reduce migraine triggers and support better brain resilience. In the previous chapter, we discussed the Mediterranean, DASH, and MIND diets as examples of two dietary patterns associated with potential benefits for brain health and migraine prevention.

Complementary Therapies

Complementary therapies for headaches offer a broad spectrum of relief, especially for those seeking non-medical alternatives. Exploring beyond traditional care can be both empowering and enlightening, presenting opportunities for individuals to take an active role in their health management.

When we talk about complementary therapies, it's essential to understand that everyone's body reacts differently to various treatments. However, diving into this realm with an open mind and a willingness to listen to your body's needs can make a significant difference.

Beyond diet and supplements, lifestyle factors like chronic stress can throw a metabolic wrench in the migraine works by dysregulating everything from inflammation to energy utilization. That's where mind-body practices come in handy. Yoga, meditation, and breathing exercises are scientifically backed methods for restoring physiological chill and metabolic equilibrium that could mean fewer migraines. Refer back to Chapter 5 where we had an in-depth discussion with practical examples for implementation.

Other commonly recognized therapies include practices like acupuncture, massage, and biofeedback, and dietary adjustments (as we just discussed), each bringing unique benefits.

Acupuncture, for instance, has ancient roots in traditional Chinese medicine and has been increasingly validated by modern research. Through the practice of inserting fine needles into specific points on the body, acupuncture is thought to balance the flow of energy—or "qi"—and alleviate pain. Some studies suggest it can be as effective as conventional treatments for certain types of chronic pain, including migraines. However, effectiveness can vary, so it's crucial to consult with a certified practitioner to see if it's the right fit for you.

Massage therapy also holds promise for migraine sufferers. Stress and tension often contribute to the frequency and severity of migraines. Regular massage sessions can help relieve muscular tension and promote relaxation, which in turn may reduce migraine episodes. Specific techniques, like trigger point therapy, target muscle knots that could be inducing referred pain in the head. In the Bonus chapter, we will discuss some useful apps and resources to assist you with these complementary therapies.

Biofeedback is another innovative tool in the complementary therapies toolkit. This involves using electronic devices to teach individuals how to control physiological functions, such as muscle tension and heart rate, which can influence headaches. Over time, patients can learn how to modulate these physical responses without equipment, offering long-term benefits.

Incorporating these natural solutions is meaningful when backed by enough evidence from the field of holistic health. Here's what you can do to approach this wisely:

- Keep a headache diary to track your symptoms, triggers, and any complementary therapies you decide to try. We will talk more about keeping track in the Bonus Chapter, where we'll explore practical tools.

- Consider consulting with healthcare providers who specialize in conventional and holistic therapies for personalized guidance.

- Start with one therapy at a time to monitor its effectiveness without the interference of other variables.

- Remain patient and consistent; complementary therapies often require a longer timeframe to demonstrate their full benefits.

Integrating these therapies into your routine should reflect a broader strategy that respects personal responsibility and the need for a safety net. Sometimes, despite our best efforts, headaches will persist. It's okay to seek help and use the tools available to us, whether they come from traditional medicine or alternative practices.

Ultimately, the goal is to tailor a multifaceted approach that combines the best of both worlds. In doing so, you address the metabolic factors and inherent complexities of headaches, and advocate for a more evidence-driven, personalized method of care. As we navigate the polarized landscape of healthcare options, the synergy between individual freedom in choosing treatments and social responsibility in promoting effective, validated practices is paramount.

Complementary therapies offer an accessible, often low-risk avenue to explore, promising relief where traditional methods may fall short. And remember, every step toward understanding and integrating these therapies is a step toward reclaiming control over your health and well-being.

Physical Activity and Weight Management

In the healthy mind-body approach, let's not forget physical activity and weight management, which was covered in more detail in Chapter 3.

Getting that body moving and shedding excess pounds does wonders for optimizing insulin resistance, cholesterol profiles, and all those other metabolic spheres linked to migraines. You don't have to run marathons, either—moderate workouts, strength training, and mindful movements like yoga or tai chi can all supply migraine-protective benefits.

Layering these holistic, natural, evidence-informed approaches alongside your traditional treatment plan is a powerful move for reclaiming control over metabolic mayhem and breaking the migraine cycle. It's about exploring all the tools in your arsenal to find what works best for *you*.

The key is to work closely with your healthcare team to develop an integrative strategy that melds pharmaceuticals with complementary, personalized lifestyle adjustments. With some metabolic fine-tuning, you may find that your migraines become a lot more manageable—and your quality of life skyrockets.

Key Takeaways

- **Unlocking metabolic health to prevent migraines:** Maintaining stable blood sugar levels, achieving a healthy weight, managing stress, ensuring adequate sleep and hydration, and balancing electrolytes help you to balance your metabolic health and prevent migraines.

- **Dietary changes play an important part in your migraine relief journey:** Following a Mediterranean diet, taking supplements such as magnesium, and trying therapies like yoga, acupuncture, and massage, can complement traditional migraine treatments effectively.

- **Balancing medicine with other holistic approaches:** Combining medications with personalized lifestyle modifications, guided by healthcare professionals, offers a comprehensive approach to managing migraines.

- **Regular physical activity and weight management:** These strategies are vital in further assisting you to improve your metabolic health and lower your risk of migraines.

To help us manage our migraines, we need to understand how metabolic factors play a role in starting and worsening these headaches. If you're interested in exploring this topic in greater depth, I have some relevant books on glucose and metabolic health as part of the Brain Health series.

For those interested, please see the appendix for more details. In the upcoming books, I offer a comprehensive examination of how metabolic dysregulation can impact brain health, delving into the latest research on mitochondrial dysfunction, insulin resistance, oxidative stress, and other metabolic pathways relevant for brain health.

*****

In the upcoming Bonus Chapter, we will explore practical tools and strategies to manage and lessen the burden of migraines and other headaches.

Chapter 9:

Bonus Chapter—Practical Tools and Resources

In this chapter, I aim to provide you with practical tools and resources to help mitigate your migraine episodes. Remember that it's a suboptimal approach to only temporarily improve your self-care because you're sick. That's like sticking a band-aid on an open wound. You're treating the symptom, not the root cause. With tools to help you manage your lifestyle consistently, you can manage your migraines throughout your life.

Building Support for Effective Migraine Management

Managing migraines can be a challenging journey, but there are many resources, applications, and solutions available to help you navigate it more effectively.

Educational Resources and Reading Materials

One of the first steps is to educate yourself about migraines, their triggers, and various management strategies. Here are some suggestions for opportunities to learn more:

- **Books and publications:** Many excellent books written by medical professionals and migraine specialists provide in-depth information about migraines, their causes, and treatment options that you may want to explore.

- **Online resources:** Reputable websites like the American Migraine Foundation, the Migraine Trust, the National Migraine Centre, and the National Headache Foundation offer a wealth of information, including educational materials, research updates, and practical tips for managing migraines.

- **Podcasts and webinars:** Listening to podcasts or attending webinars hosted by migraine experts can be a convenient way to learn more about the latest developments and strategies in migraine management.

- **Join my mailing list:** If you're interested in periodically receiving more information, including tips for improving migraines, and regular free live webinars, I would like to invite you to subscribe to my mailing list. To join, follow the QR code provided at the end of this book, or the link bit.ly/migraine-book-bonuses

Building a Supportive Migraine Community

As you embark on implementing lifestyle changes and new management strategies, having a supportive community can be invaluable. Connecting with others who understand the challenges of living with migraines can provide encouragement, motivation, and a sense of belonging.

- **Online support groups:** There are various online forums and social media groups dedicated to migraine support, where you can connect with others, share experiences, and offer or receive advice.

- **In-person support groups:** Many cities have in-person support groups for individuals with migraines, which can be a great way to connect with others in your area.

- **Advocacy organizations:** These are organizations like Miles for Migraine and the Coalition for Headache and Migraine Patients (CHAMP), which offer opportunities to get involved in advocacy efforts and connect with the migraine community.

- **Online programs and resources:** In addition to support groups, there are various online resources and communities dedicated to migraine management. For example, the Canadian

Headache Society offers the Mastermind program that offers educational resources, and personalized guidance for implementing lifestyle changes and managing migraines effectively. I also offer an online Migraine-free BRA(i)NS® mentorship program, see appendix for information if of interest.

Personalizing Your Migraine Management Approach

It's important to remember that every individual is unique—what works for one person may not work for another. This is also true when it comes to managing your migraines.

- **Identifying your triggers:** We've already discussed how important is it to keep a detailed migraine diary for tracking potential triggers, such as specific foods, stress levels, sleep patterns, or environmental factors.

- **Experimenting and adjusting strategies:** Be open to trying different strategies and making adjustments based on your personal experiences and choices.

- **Seeking professional guidance:** Work with your healthcare provider or a migraine specialist to develop a personalized plan that takes into account your unique needs and circumstances.

- **Finding the right strategies for you:** Remember, the key to successful migraine management is finding the strategies that work best for you. Don't be discouraged if it takes time and experimentation to find the right approach. Stay patient, stay persistent, and don't hesitate to reach out for support.

Let's delve a little deeper into these different strategies that you may decide to employ on your journey.

Migraine Tracking and Trigger Identification

The more you can crack the code of your unique migraine puzzle through meticulous tracking, the better armed you'll be to tackle triggers head-on and prevent future brain battles. It's the first major step in reclaiming control over this debilitating condition.

The Importance of Keeping a Detailed Migraine Journal

Remember my comparison in Chapter 7 (when discussing keeping a food diary) between keeping a detailed migraine diary and being a detective investigating your migraine mystery? Well, this concept also applies to other lifestyle habits. Think about it—migraines can be incredibly personal and what sets one person's migraine cycle into motion might be different for the next person. That's why tracking your symptoms and potential triggers is so important.

It's all about connecting the dots and looking for patterns. Was that brutal migraine triggered by the red wine you had with your dinner last night? Or was it all the stress at work? Are you experiencing hormonal changes? By diligently recording details about what you ate, how you slept, your cycle, and major events or emotions, you start piecing together your own personal pie chart of migraine triggers.

And having all that data on hand makes your next doctor's appointment way more high-value. Instead of just vague recollections, you can whip out your migraine dossier and give your provider a clear window into your experiences. That makes it easier for them to develop an effective, personalized treatment plan catered specifically to your needs.

- **Emotional release:** When you feel the beginnings of a migraine aura or that tight pain starting to grip your head, immediately grab your journal. Then do a brain dump, venting all your feelings onto the page without censorship. Getting out that emotional turmoil prevents it from staying bottled up and manifesting physical pain.

- **Cognitive restructuring:** During an attack, negative thought spirals are common. You may catch yourself thinking things like "I'll never get relief," "I'm disabled by this," and more. Journaling helps inject some rational perspective. Re-read earlier entries about getting through past episodes and re-frame your mindset from one of despair to patient perseverance.

- **Creative expression:** Whether it's free-form poetry, sketching your pain patterns, or calligraphy mantras, being creatively expressive is so therapeutic. Making something beautiful out of something difficult is empowering. Your migraine-inspired art can be very cathartic.

- **Gratitude practice:** On good days, make lists of what you're grateful for—being able to prepare a meal, play with your dog, or just breathe fresh air. This positivity primes your mindset for resilience during inevitable tough episodes.

The act of writing things down is almost like lancing a pressure valve in your mind and body, clearing out the backlog of emotional gunk that often exacerbates and prolongs migraine attacks.

Take your trusty journal everywhere with you. This will give you an outlet to proactively maintain your emotional, mental, and physical wellness. It's an affordable, versatile tool for your migraine coping toolkit.

Recording Potential Triggers

When trying to identify potential migraine triggers, consider tracking everything from the foods you nibble to the storms brewing outside. Your journal functions as a migraine diary. Note down things like your food intake, sleep quality, menstrual cycle, stress levels, weather changes—anything that could be a potential trigger. Over time, patterns emerge that allow you to be proactive about prevention.

In Chapter 7, we established that food is a huge one—certain ingredients or additives can be crazy migraine instigators for some people. By jotting down your full menu, you may notice head-splitting patterns emerging after that anchovy pizza or pile of aged cheese. Once identified, you can kiss those culinary culprits goodbye.

But it's not just about what you eat. Hormonal ups and downs for women can prime the migraine firing squad. Carefully logging your menstrual cycles and details around peri-menopause or menopause gives clues into these biochemical domino effects.

Stress is another big, bad migraine catalyst, so taking note of any work crunches, family pressures, or just general life chaos pays off. You may see migraines cluster around your most maxed-out weeks.

Then there are external forces, like the wildcard weather. Radical shifts in temperatures, humidity, or even air pressure and storm fronts can potentially push some people's migraine buttons. Tracking Mother Nature's mood swings helps reveal her influence.

While documentation can be helpful, it's important to approach it with balance and an open mind, as even subtle lifestyle factors or patterns may provide insights into managing your unique migraine experience.

Apps and Digital Tools for Easy Migraine Tracking

The beauty of modern technology is there are tons of user-friendly apps and digital tools designed to make militant migraine tracking a total breeze. You can quickly log details from your smartphone in just a few taps. Heck, some apps even allow you to snap pics of your migraine meds or scan barcodes on your food packages! Here are some apps and digital tools that can make tracking easier:

- **Migraine Buddy:** This app allows you to track your migraines, including symptoms, triggers, and medications. It also provides insights and reports to help you understand your migraine patterns.

- **N1–Headaches Curelator App:** This app helps you track your migraines, symptoms, and potential triggers. It also offers personalized insights based on your data to help you manage your migraines more effectively.

- **Migraine Monitor:** Keeps a record of your migraines by monitoring your triggers, symptoms, and treatments. It also provides customizable reports to share with your healthcare provider.

- **iHeadache:** This app allows you to track your migraines, including pain intensity, triggers, and medications. It also offers personalized reports to help you identify patterns and triggers.

Using these apps and tools can help you track your migraines more easily and provide valuable information that you and your healthcare provider can use to manage your migraines effectively.

Using the Information in Conjunction With Your Doctor

Work closely with your doctor to identify your migraine triggers. The results from your journal or app will help your doctor a lot. They can help you analyze your symptoms, lifestyle factors, and potential triggers to pinpoint patterns. Together, you can develop a plan to manage your migraines and minimize their impact on your life.

Tools for Complementary and Integrative Therapies

Here are some practical apps and other resources for managing migraines through complementary and integrative therapies. Many of these are free or have free versions, work on both iOS/Android, and allow you to customize therapies or get guidance for migraine relief on the go.

Helpful Resources for Holistic Migraine Management

Integrating complementary therapies into your migraine management plan can provide additional support and help you take a holistic approach to your health and well-being.

Massage, Acupressure, and Acupuncture Apps

Regular massage therapy can help reduce muscle tension and stress. Acupuncture may help lessen the frequency and severity of migraines. Some of the apps you may want to explore, are:

- **Massage Rebel (iOS, Android):** This app provides guided massage routines specifically designed for relieving headaches and migraines. It includes techniques like temple massages, pressure point therapy, and neck/shoulder massage routines.

- **Headache Relief Massage (Android):** This app is focused on self-massage for headache and migraine relief. It has visual guides and instructions for acupressure points as well as neck, scalp, and facial massage techniques.

- **Migraine Massage Buddy (iOS):** Created by a massage therapist, this app demonstrates massage techniques like effleurage, petrissage, and trigger point therapy to relieve migraine pain. It has timers and reminders.

- **Apps for acupuncture and acupressure:** Simple Acupressure and Acupuncture Mate.

Using an app can make it more convenient to regularly practice acupressure, which some find helpful for migraine prevention and management between acute attacks.

Aromatherapy Apps

Essential oils like lavender or peppermint could potentially reduce migraine symptoms. You can inhale these oils or apply them to your skin (diluted with a carrier oil) for relief. Apps to help you personalize your essential oil blends, combine your blends with the use of music, and see consumer ratings for existing blends, include:

- Revive

- Essence

- AromaTrail

Apps for Mind-Body Approaches

Practices like yoga, tai chi, and biofeedback can help manage stress and improve overall well-being, which may reduce the frequency and severity of migraines. Meditation and mindfulness are other great ways to focus on specific areas of your body and help you to relax. Meditation or mindfulness apps to consider are:

- **Ten Percent Happier:** Offering expert coaching on stress reduction and meditation (sign up for a bonus discount using the link in the Appendix)

- **Calm:** Guided meditation, sleep stories, mindfulness exercises

- **Headspace:** Meditation and mindfulness training

- **Insight Timer:** Thousands of free guided meditations

Yoga or Exercise Apps to consider are:

- **Down Dog:** Customized yoga practice videos

- **Nike Training Club:** Free workouts, yoga, mindfulness

- **Alo Moves:** Yoga, meditation, and other fitness classes

Apps About Oral Supplements and Herbs

You might remember we discussed some of these apps earlier in the book. Some people find relief from migraines by taking certain supplements or herbs, such as magnesium, riboflavin (vitamin B2), feverfew, or butterbur. Supplement or Herb Tracker Apps, include:

- **MyFitnessPal:** Log supplements, herbs, and track nutrients

- **Youtrition:** Reminders and tracking for vitamins/supplements

Evidence-Based Practice Resources

Explore therapies that have scientific evidence supporting their effectiveness for migraines. Websites such as the National Center for Complementary and Integrative Health (NCCIH) and the Cochrane Library offer trustworthy information regarding the effectiveness of various therapies.

Tips for Adjusting Your Environment

Migraine management often involves making environmental adjustments to reduce exposure to potential triggers and create a more comfortable space during attacks. Here are some practical tools and resources for managing environmental factors.

Low-Stimulus Environments During Migraine Attacks

- Create a dark, quiet, and cool room by closing curtains or blinds, turning off lights, and using a fan or air conditioner.

- Minimize noise by using earplugs or noise-cancelling headphones.

- Avoid strong smells, such as perfumes, cleaning products, or certain foods.

Managing light, sound, and smell triggers

- Use light-filtering or blackout curtains to control light exposure.

- Install dimmer switches or use lamps with adjustable brightness.

- Use white noise machines or apps to mask external sounds.

- Consider using air purifiers or essential oil diffusers (with caution) to manage odors.

Using sunglasses, noise-cancelling devices, and essential oils

- Invest in a good pair of sunglasses or migraine glasses with tinted lenses to reduce light sensitivity.

- Use noise-canceling headphones or earplugs to block out loud noises.

- Explore essential oils like peppermint or lavender, which may provide relief for some individuals (use caution and consult your healthcare professional).

Creating a personalized migraine-friendly space

- Designate a quiet, dark room or area in your home as a migraine retreat.

- Use blackout curtains, soundproofing materials, and comfortable bedding to create a soothing environment.

- Keep a migraine toolkit nearby with items like ice packs, eye masks, earplugs, and any necessary medications.

- Consider using calming scents, soft lighting, or white noise machines to personalize the space.

Remember, everyone's migraine triggers and lifestyle choices will differ, so it's important to experiment and find the environmental adjustments that work best for you. Consulting with a healthcare professional or migraine specialist can also help you develop a comprehensive migraine management plan.

Key Takeaways

- **Managing migraines requires a multifaceted approach:** This involves lifestyle modifications, dietary changes, stress management techniques, and environmental adjustments.

- **Incorporating practical tools and resources into your daily routine:** This can help you manage migraines and improve your overall quality of life. A variety of apps and online resources are available to assist you on your wellness journey.

- **Personalization is key:** What works for one person may not work for another. Work closely with healthcare providers to find the best treatment plan tailored to your specific needs.

- **Foster resilience and self-efficacy:** By doing this you take control of your migraine management and navigate challenges with confidence.

*****

Now that we've reached the end of this incredible learning experience, let's briefly recap by concluding what we've learned so far as we look forward to the path ahead.

Conclusion

In *Break Free From Migraines Naturally*, we focused on the power of your lifestyle and taking a comprehensive, holistic approach to managing your migraines. Our primary focus was on preventative strategies that go beyond just treating symptoms, and holistically treating your current symptoms.

You see, each of us has a threshold for migraines—an invisible line that, when crossed, increases the likelihood of an attack occurring. It's almost like a scale, with various triggers piling up on one side until they outweigh your body's ability to counterbalance them. My mission here is to help you raise that threshold as high as possible, fortifying your resilience so you can better withstand life's stresses without toppling into a migraine.

We've tackled this in two main ways: By nurturing your brain resilience, and by restoring balance to your autonomic nervous system (ANS)—the control center that regulates key bodily functions. I also deliver this approach of building brain resilience and balancing your autonomic nervous system, through the BRA(i)NS® program (see appendix for details).

I understand how overwhelming migraines can feel, which is why my approach aims to meet you where you are. I hope this has been a journey of transformation for you up to now. Even more, I hope you will continue with this journey, and see it through to better, pain-free days.

Final Thoughts

Throughout the book, we've explored a holistic approach to migraine management that goes beyond treating symptoms. By nurturing brain resilience through optimizing sleep, physical activity, nutrition, supplements, metabolic health, and gut-brain health, you're equipping your body and mind with the tools to withstand migraine triggers more effectively.

Restoring balance to your ANS through mindfulness, breathwork, yoga, and mind-body practices further fortifies your ability to counteract the stresses that can precipitate migraine attacks. And by understanding the roles of hormones, incorporating complementary therapies, and developing strategies to identify and avoid personal triggers, you're taking the first steps toward raising your migraine threshold.

This journey toward migraine relief is not a quick fix, but a lifestyle transformation that requires patience, commitment, and self-compassion. There may be setbacks along the way, but by consistently implementing the strategies outlined in this book, you're laying a strong foundation for long-term migraine management.

Remember, you're not alone in this battle. Countless others have walked this path before you, and by sharing our collective wisdom and experiences, we can support one another in reclaiming our lives from the grip of migraines.

I encourage you to persevere with the strategies and insights shared in this book, adapting and refining your approach as needed. Migraine management is an ongoing journey, but one that is well worth the effort for the invaluable gift of living a life free from the relentless pain and disruption of these debilitating attacks.

Now, I am kindly asking you for a moment of your time. If you found value in the insights, strategies, and knowledge shared in this book, I would be incredibly grateful if you could take a few minutes to leave a review. Your honest thoughts and feedback are invaluable to me, and I intend to read every single review with care and appreciation.

Not only do reader reviews inspire me to continue creating meaningful content, but they also help fellow readers make informed decisions about their next reading choices. A review, no matter how brief, is a small gesture that can make a profound impact. Your support means the world to me, and I thank you in advance for considering this request.

If you want to stay in touch and receive news about upcoming workshops and events regarding brain health matters. I regularly offer free migraine webinars, so I encourage you to sign up for my mailing list at bit.ly/drwongbrainhealth to stay informed about upcoming events. You will also find a QR code at the end of this book to direct you to my website. Keep an eye out for my next books, including *The Brain Health Book for Adults*, in which I will be sharing practical steps for improved brain health, such as achieving clarity and focus.

*****

I wish you all the best on this transformative path, and I hope this book serves as a trusted guide and source of empowerment along the way.

Can you help please?

Thank you again for reading this book! I hope you've found this interesting & helpful.

Book reviews make all the difference in the discoverability of books.

I would love to hear your thoughts with a quick review on Amazon.

I deeply appreciate this and will read your reviews.

For your convenience, the following QR codes or links take you to directly to the review page at your respective Amazon marketplace:

Amazon.com	Amazon.ca
Amazon.com/review/create-review?&asin= 1738558169	Amazon.ca/review/create-review?&asin= 1738558169
Amazon.co.uk	Amazon.com.au
Amazon.co.uk/review/create-review?&asin= 1738558169	Amazon.com.au/review/create-review?&asin= 1738558169

Amazon.de/review/create-review?&asin=1738558169
Amazon.fr/review/create-review?&asin= 1738558169
Amazon.es/review/create-review?&asin= 1738558169
Amazon.it/review/create-review?&asin= 1738558169
Amazon.nl/review/create-review?&asin= 1738558169
Amazon.se/review/create-review?&asin= 1738558169
Amazon.pl/review/create-review?&asin= 1738558169
Amazon.sg/review/create-review?&asin= 1738558169

Appendix

Would you like to join one of my upcoming Migraine-free BRA(i)NS ® webinars for FREE?

Receive your migraine book bonuses, which include:

- Self-massage & soft-tissue guide for Migraine relief
- Sleep Checklist
- Mindfulness Meditation audioguides
- A free ticket to my Migraine-free BRA(i)NS ® webinar
- Discount for the 10% Happier meditation app

Register for your bonuses using this link

bit.ly/migraine-book-bonuses

Would you like a free Kindle copy of one of my upcoming books?

My mission with writing these books is to empower people with good quality information to improve their brain health and well-being.

Coming soon:

Magnesium: Restore and Revitalize Your Brain and Body

Sleep Better to Thrive: Practical Steps That Will Enhance Your Life

Quit Ultra-processed Foods Now: Practical Steps to Transform Your Lifestyle and Feel Better Fast

Register your interest here:

bit.ly/drwongbooks

References

The references provided below include a mixture of scientific articles and educational websites that provide valuable information and that you can easily access to do further reading. Keep in mind that new studies are constantly being conducted. You can use the resources here to help you build your knowledge base and take ownership of your health journey.

Afridi, S. K. (2018). Current concepts in migraine and their relevance to pregnancy. *Obstetric medicine, 11*(4), 154–159. https://doi.org/10.1177/1753495X18769170

Al-Hassany, L., Haas, J., Piccininni, M., Kurth, T., Maassen Van Den Brink, A., & Rohmann, J. L. (2020). Giving researchers a headache—Sex and gender differences in migraine. *Frontiers in neurology, 11,* 549038. https://doi.org/10.3389/fneur.2020.549038

American Academy of Allergies, Asthma & Immunology (AAAAI). (2023, December 27). *Allergy headaches and sinus headaches.* https://www.aaaai.org/tools-for-the-public/conditions-library/allergies/headaches-connected-to-allergies-and-sinus-problem

American Migraine Foundation. (n.d). *Migraine A-Z the things our experts want you to know.* https://americanmigrainefoundation.org/glossary/

Amin, F. M., Aristeidou, S., Baraldi, C., Czapinska-Ciepiela, E. K., Ariadni, D. D., Di Lenola, D., Fenech, C., Kampouris, K., Karagiorgis, G., Braschinsky, M., Linde, M., & European

Headache Federation School of Advanced Studies (EHF-SAS), 2018). The association between migraine and physical exercise. *The journal of headache and pain*, *19*(1), 83. https://doi.org/10.1186/s10194-018-0902-y

Amiri, P., Kazeminasab, S., Nejadghaderi, S. A., Mohammadinasab, R., Pourfathi, H., Araj-Khodaei, M., Sullman, M. J. M., Kolahi, A. A., & Safiri, S. (2022). Migraine: A review on its history, global epidemiology, risk factors, and comorbidities. *Frontiers in neurology*, *12*, 800605. https://doi.org/10.3389/fneur.2021.800605

Balban, M. Y., Neri, E., Kogon, M. M., Weed, L., Nouriani, B., Jo, B., Holl, G., Zeitzer, J. M., Spiegel, D., & Huberman, A. D. (2023). Brief structured respiration practices enhance mood and reduce physiological arousal. *Cell reports. Medicine*, *4*(1), 100895. https://doi.org/10.1016/j.xcrm.2022.100895

Barth, C., Villringer, A., & Sacher, J. (2015). Sex hormones affect neurotransmitters and shape the adult female brain during hormonal transition periods. *Frontiers in neuroscience*, *9*, 37. https://doi.org/10.3389/fnins.2015.00037

Becker, W. J. (2018). Migraine and Pregnancy. Headache: The Journal of Head and Face Pain, 58(9), 1479-1493. https://doi.org/10.1111/head.13378

Biscetti, L., Cresta, E., Cupini, L. M., Calabresi, P., Sarchielli, P. (2023). The putative role of neuroinflammation in the complex pathophysiology of migraine: From bench to bedside. *Neurobiology of disease,* 180. https://doi.org/10.1016/j.nbd.2023.106072.

Brown, B. (2022). Migraine headaches: opportunities for management with precision nutrition. *Nutritional Medicine Journal*, 1 (3), 117-152.

Calhoun, A. H. (2012). Current topics and controversies in menstrual migraine. *Headache: The journal of head and face pain*, 1 (52), 8-11. https://doi.org/10.1111/j.1526-4610.2012.02130.x

Calhoun, A. H. (2017). Migraine treatment in pregnancy and lactation. *Current Pain and Headache Reports* 21, 46. https://doi.org/10.1007/s11916-017-0646-4.

Cardia, L., Calapai, F., Mondello, C., Quattrone, D., Elisa Sorbara, E., Mannucci, C., Calapai, G., & Mondello, E. (2020). Clinical use of omega-3 fatty acids in migraine: A narrative review. *Medicine*, 99(42), e22253. https://doi.org/10.1097/MD.0000000000022253

Centers for Disease Control and Prevention (2022, September 13). https://www.cdc.gov/sleep/about_sleep/sleep_hygiene.html

Champaloux, S. W., Tepper, N. K., Monsour, M., Curtis, K. M., Whiteman, M. K., Marchbanks, P. A., & Curtin, D. (2017). Use of combined hormonal contraceptives among women with migraines and risk of ischemic stroke. *American Journal of Obstetrics and Gynecology*, 216(5), 489.e1-489.e7. https://doi.org/10.1016/j.ajog.2017.01.024

Chen, P. K., & Wang, S. J. (2018). Non-headache symptoms in migraine patients. *Research*, 7, 188. https://doi.org/10.12688/f1000research.12447.1

Chen, Q., Chen, O., Martins, I. M., Hou, H., Zhao, X., Blumberg, J. B., & Li, B. (2017). Collagen peptides ameliorate intestinal epithelial barrier dysfunction in immunostimulatory Caco-2 cell monolayers via enhancing tight junctions. *Food & function*, 8(3), 1144–1151. https://doi.org/10.1039/c6fo01347c

Cleveland Clinic. (n.d.). *Headaches.* https://my.clevelandclinic.org/health/diseases/9639-headaches

Crida, D. (n.d.). *Nutritional strategies for migraine prevention.* Igennus Healthcare Nutrition. https://igennus.com/blogs/articles/nutritional-strategies-for-migraine-prevention

Diamond, M., & Marcus, D. (2016, August 13). *Diet and headache control.* American Migraine Foundation. https://americanmigrainefoundation.org/resource-library/diet/

Dimidi, E., Cox, S. R., Rossi, M., Whelan K. Fermented Foods: Definitions and characteristics, Impact on the gut microbiota and effects on gastrointestinal health and disease. *Nutrients.* 2019; 11(8):1806. https://doi.org/10.3390/nu11081806

Edvinsson, L., Haanes, K. A., Warfvinge, K. (2019, July 1). Does inflammation have a role in migraine? *Nature Reviews Neurology,* 15 (483–490). https://doi.org/10.1038/s41582-019-0216-y

Efthymakis, C, Matteo, N. (2022). The role of Zinc L-Carnosine in the prevention and treatment of gastrointestinal mucosal disease in humans: a review. *Clinics and Research in Hepatology and Gastroenterology,* 46 (7) https://doi.org/10.1016/j.clinre.2022.101954.

Ezra, Y., & Colson, N. J. (2015). Hormone therapy and migraine. Therapy, 12(3), 339-357. https://doi.org/10.2217/pmt.15.9

Fishell, R. A. (1988). The relationship between position and incidence of spinal headache following spinal anesthesia in the young adult female. *Virginia Commonwealth University VCU Scholars Compass. Thesis and dissertations.* https://doi.org/10.25772/KGQB-1S86

Gao, L., Huanhuan, Q., Gao, N., Kai, L., Dang, E., Wenbin, T., Gang, W. (2020). A retrospective analysis for facial telangiectasia treatment using pulsed dye laser and intense pulsed light configured with different wavelength bands. *J Cosmet Dermatol.* 2020; 19: 88–92. https://doi.org/10.1111/jocd.13179

Garza, I. & Schwedt, T. J. (2023, Jan 17). *Hemicrania continua.* UptoDate. https://www.uptodate.com/contents/hemicrania-continua

Genetics, pathophysiology, diagnosis, treatment, management, and prevention of migraine. *Journal of neurology* https://www.sciencedirect.com/science/article/pii/S07533322 21003425

Goadsby, P. (n.d). *Quote by Dr Peter Goadsby in What is a migraine?* The Migraine Trust. https://migrainetrust.org/understand-migraine/what-is-migraine/

Goadsby, P. J. (2021, October 18). Recognize the non-headache symptoms of migraines. UCLA Health. https://www.uclahealth.org/news/migraine-non-headache-symptoms

Goadsby, P. J., Holland, P. R., Martins-Oliveira, M., Hoffmann, J., Schankin, C., & Akerman, S. (2017). Pathophysiology of Migraine: A Disorder of Sensory Processing. *Physiological reviews*, *97*(2), 553–622. https://doi.org/10.1152/physrev.00034.2015

Gross, E. C., Klement, R. J., Schoenen, J., D'Agostino, D. P., & Fischer, D. (2019). Potential protective mechanisms of ketone bodies in migraine prevention. *Nutrients*, *11*(4), 811. https://doi.org/10.3390/nu11040811

Harvard Health Publishing (n.d.). *Sleep*. https://www.health.harvard.edu/topics/sleep

Harvard Health Publishing. (2023, June 13). *What your heart rate is telling you*. Harvard Medical School. https://www.health.harvard.edu/heart-health/what-your-heart-rate-is-telling-you

Healthdirect (n.d.). *Migraine*. https://www.healthdirect.gov.au/migraine

Hindiyeh, N. A., Zhang, N., Farrar, M., Banerjee, P., Lombard, L., & Aurora, S. K. (2020). The role of diet and nutrition in migraine triggers and treatment: A systematic literature review. *Headache: The Journal of Head and Face Pain*, *60*(7), 1300–1316. https://doi.org/10.1111/head.13836

Holroyd, K. A., Cottrell, C. K., Rios Riesgo, D., Hodges, A., Penzien, D., Chase, D., ... & Lipchik, G. L. (2020). Interdisciplinary management of migraine: a clinical guide for headache providers. *Canadian Journal of Neurological Sciences*, 47(6), 710-732. https://doi.org/10.1017/cjn.2020.138

Jenny. (2023, November 17). *Nutrition and migraine relief: What to eat and avoid*. Migraine Buddy. https://migrainebuddy.com/nutrition-and-migraine-relief-what-to-eat-and-avoid/

John Hopkins Medicine (n.d.). *Vestibular migraine*. https://www.hopkinsmedicine.org/health/conditions-and-diseases/vestibular-migraine

Jovel, E. C. A. , & Mejía, S. F. E. (2017). Caffeine and headache: specific remarks. *Neurología*, *32*(6), 394–398. https://doi.org/10.1016/j.nrl.2014.12.016

Kissoon, N. R., Steel, S. (2023). *Patient education: Headache treatment in adults (Beyond the Basics)*. UpToDate. https://www.uptodate.com/contents/headache-treatment-in-adults-beyond-the-basics

Kissoon, N. R., Steel, S. (2023, March 24). Up to Date. https://www.uptodate.com/contents/migraines-in-adults-beyond-the-basics

Koppen, H., & van Veldhoven, P. L. (2013). Migraineurs with exercise-triggered attacks have a distinct migraine. *The journal of headache and pain*, *14*(1), 99. https://doi.org/10.1186/1129-2377-14-99

Kuruvilla, D. (2018, November 29). *Holistic treatments for migraine.* American Migraine Foundation. https://americanmigrainefoundation.org/resource-library/holistic-treatments-for-migraine/

Kuruvilla, D. E., Mehta, A., Ravishankar, N. and Cowan, R.P. (2021). A patient perspective of complementary and integrative medicine (CIM) for migraine treatment: a social media survey. *BMC complementary medicine and therapies*, 21(1). https://doi.org/10.1186/s12906-021-03226-0.

Kvisvik, E. V., Stovner, L. J., Helde, G., Bovim, G., & Linde, M. (2011). Headache and migraine during pregnancy and puerperium: the MIGRA-study. The Journal of Headache and Pain, 12(4), 443-451. https://doi.org/10.1007/s10194-011-0329-1

Lemmens, J., De Pauw, J., Van Soom, T., Michiels, S., Versijpt, J., van Breda, E., Castien, R. & De Hertogh, W. (2019). The effect of aerobic exercise on the number of migraine days, duration and pain intensity in migraine: a systematic literature review and meta-analysis. *The journal of headache and pain*, 20(1). https://doi.org/10.1186/s10194-019-0961-8.

Levy, J. (2021, March 4). *Marshmallow root: The ultimate gut and lung protector.* Draxe.com. https://draxe.com/nutrition/marshmallow-root/

Lindberg, S. (2021, *Does exercise help migraine relief? What research shows.* Healthline. https://www.healthline.com/health/migraine/does-exercise-help-migraines

Lopp, S., Navidi, W., Achermann, P., LeBourgeois, M., & Diniz Behn, C. (2017). Developmental Changes in Ultradian Sleep Cycles across Early Childhood. Journal of biological rhythms, 32(1), 64–74. https://doi.org/10.1177/0748730416685451

MacGregor, E. A., Frith, A., Ellis, J., Aspinall, L., & Hackshaw, A. (2010). Incidence of migraine relative to menstrual cycle phases of rising and falling estrogen. Neurology, 67(12), 2154-2158. https://doi.org/10.1212/01.wnl.0000233888.18228.19

Martami. F., Togha, M., Seifishahpar, M., Ghorbani, Z., Ansari, H., Karimi, T., Jahromi, S. R. (2019). The effects of a multispecies probiotic supplement on inflammatory markers and episodic and chronic migraine characteristics: A randomized double-blind controlled trial. *Cephalalgia*;39(7): 841-853. https://doi.org/10.1177/0333102418820102

Mavroudis, I., Ciobica, A., Luca, A. C., & Balmus, I. M. (2023). Post-Traumatic Headache: A Review of Prevalence, Clinical Features, Risk Factors, and Treatment Strategies. *Journal of clinical medicine*, *12*(13), 4233. https://doi.org/10.3390/jcm12134233

Migraine Research Foundation (n.d.). *Migraine facts*. https://migraineresearchfoundation.org/about-migraine/migraine-facts/

Migraine Headache published in the National Library of Medicine https://www.ncbi.nlm.nih.gov/books/NBK560787/

Migraine: from pathophysiology to treatment" published in the Journal of   Neurology https://link.springer.com/article/10.1007/s00415-023-11706-1

The Migraine Trust. (n.d–a). *Migraine and sleep.* https://migrainetrust.org/live-with-migraine/self-management/migraine-and-sleep/

The Migraine Trust. (n.d–b). *Supplements.* https://migrainetrust.org/live-with-migraine/healthcare/treatments/supplements/

Mungoven, T. J., Henderson, L. A., Meylakh, N. (2021). Chronic migraine pathophysiology and treatment: A review of current perspectives. Frontiers in Pain Research, 2. https://doi.org/10.3389/fpain.2021.705276

Nowaczewska, M., Wiciński, M., Kaźmierczak, W. *The ambiguous role of caffeine in migraine headache: From trigger to treatment. Nutrients.* 2020; 12(8):2259. https://doi.org/10.3390/nu12082259

Myers, A. (n.d). Restore gut health with 6 herbs and nutrients. https://www.amymyersmd.com/article/restore-gut-health-herbs-nutrients

Namazi, N., Heshmati, J., & Tarighat-Esfanjani, A. (2015). Supplementation with riboflavin (vitamin B2) for migraine prophylaxis in adults and children: A review. *International journal for vitamin and nutrition research. Internationale Zeitschrift für Vitamin-und Ernahrungsforschung. Journal international de vitaminologie et de nutrition, 85*(1-2), 79–87. https://doi.org/10.1024/0300-9831/a000225

Nappi, R.E., Sances, G., Detaddei, S., Ornati, A., Polatti, F., & Náppi, G. (2009). Hormonal management of migraine at menopause. *Menopause International,* 15(2), 82-86. https://doi.org/10.1258/mi.2009.009019

National Heart, Blood and Lung Institute. (2022, March 24). *Sleep phases and stages.* https://www.nhlbi.nih.gov/health/sleep/stages-of-sleep

National Institute for Health and Care Excellence (NICE). (n.d.). *NICE Clinical Knowledge Summaries (CKS).* https://www.nice.org.uk/

NHS Health Scotland. (2023, January 4). *Health benefits of eating well.* NHS Inform. https://www.nhsinform.scot/healthy-living/food-and-nutrition/eating-well/health-benefits-of-eating-well/

NHS. (2022, July 29). *Eating a balanced diet.* https://www.nhs.uk/live-well/eat-well/how-to-eat-a-balanced-diet/eating-a-balanced-diet/

NICE. (2012). *Recommendations: Headaches in over 12s: Diagnosis and management.* https://www.nice.org.uk/guidance/cg150/chapter/Recommendations

The Nutrition Source. (n.d.). *Diet review: DASH.* Harvard T.H. Chan School of Public Health. https://nutritionsource.hsph.harvard.edu/healthy-weight/diet-reviews/dash-diet/

Pacheco, D., & Singh, A. (2023, November 3). *What is NREM sleep?* Sleep Foundation. *https://www.sleepfoundation.org/stages-of-sleep/nrem-sleep*

Pavlović, J. M., Allshouse, A. A., Santoro, N. F., Crawford, S. L., Thurston, R. C., Neal-Perry, G. S., & Derby, C. A. (2014). Influence of regular menstrual cycle and age on hormone derivative levels in the Follicular phase of the menstrual cycle. *Menopause*, 21(6), 612-620. https://doi.org/10.1097/GME.0b013e3182a80cf8

Pavlović, J. M., Allshouse, A. A., Santoro, N. F., Crawford, S. L., Thurston, R. C., Neal-Perry, G. S., Lipton, R. B., & Derby, C. A. (2016). Sex hormones in women with and without migraine: Evidence of migraine-specific hormone profiles. *Neurology*, 87(1), 49–56. https://doi.org/10.1212/WNL.0000000000002798

Pearson, K., Burford, M. (2023, April 21). *The MIND diet: A detailed guide for beginners.* Healthline. https://www.healthline.com/nutrition/mind-diet

Poulsen, A. H., Younis, S., Thuraiaiyah, J. & Ashina, M. (2021). The chronobiology of migraine: a systematic review. The *journal of headache and pain* 22, 76. https://doi.org/10.1186/s10194-021-01276-w

Reddy, S., Reddy V., & Sharma, S. (2023, May 1). *Physiology, circadian rhythm.* StatPearls Publishing. https://www.ncbi.nlm.nih.gov/books/NBK519507/

Ripa, P., Ornello, R., Degan, D., Tiseo, C., Stewart, J., Pistoia, F., &

Sacco, S. (2015). Migraine in menopausal women: a systematic review. *International journal of women's health*, 7, 773-782. https://doi.org/10.2147/IJWH.S70073

Rizzoli, P. (2022, February 15). Health disparities and headache treatment. *Harvard Health Publishing Blog*. Harvard Medical School. https://www.health.harvard.edu/blog/health-disparities-and-headache-treatment-202202152685

RocketEditor. (2022, July 19). Silent migraines: Definition & symptoms. *Brain Center Blog*. https://braincenter.org/2022/07/19/silent-migraines-definition-symptoms/

Sances, G., Granella, F., Nappi, R. E., Fignon, A., Ghiotto, N., Polatti, F., & Nappi, G. (2003). Course of migraine during pregnancy and postpartum: a prospective study. *Cephalalgia*, 23(3), 197-205. https://doi.org/10.1046/j.1468-2982.2003.00480.x

Singh, N. N., & Sahota, P. (2013). Sleep-related headache and its management. *Current treatment options in neurology*, 15(6), 704–722. https://doi.org/10.1007/s11940-013-0258-1

Soveyd, N., Abdolahi, M., Bitarafan, S., Tafakhori, A., Sarraf, P., Togha, M., Okhovat, A. A., Hatami, M., Sedighiyan, M., Djalali, M., & Mohammadzadeh Honarvar, N. (2017). Molecular mechanisms of omega-3 fatty acids in the migraine headache. *Iranian journal of neurology*, 16(4), 210–217. https://www.ncbi.nlm.nih.gov/pmc/articles/PMC5937007/

Spekker, E., & Nagy-Grócz, G. (2023). All roads lead to the gut: The importance of the microbiota and diet in migraine. *Neurology*

international, 15(3), 1174–1190.
https://doi.org/10.3390/neurolint15030073

Stages of a migraine attack (n.d.). The Migraine Trust.
https://migrainetrust.org/understand-migraine/

Stanford Online. (n.d.). *Course: An evidence-based approach to the diagnosis and management of migraines in adults in the primary care and general neurology setting.* Stanford School of Medicine.
https://online.stanford.edu/courses/som-ycme0039-evidence-based-approach-diagnosis-and-management-migraines-adults-primary-care

Stibich, M. (2023, May 18). *10 benefits of sleep.* Verywell Health.
https://www.verywellhealth.com/top-health-benefits-of-a-good-nights-sleep-2223766

Stovner, L.J., Hagen, K., Linde, M., Steiner, T., J. (2022). The global prevalence of headache: an update, with analysis of the influences of methodological factors on prevalence estimates. *Journal of Headache Pain,* 23 (34).
https://doi.org/10.1186/s10194-022-01402-2

Summer, J., & Wright, H. (2023). *Hypnic headaches.* Sleep Foundation.
https://www.sleepfoundation.org/physical-health/hypnic-headaches

Sweet, J. (2024, January 4). *Master your sleep schedule: Best tips for a healthy routine.* Sleep.com https://www.sleep.com/sleep-health/sleep-schedule

Varkey, E., Cider, A., Carlsson, J., & Linde, M. (2011). Exercise as migraine prophylaxis: a randomized study using relaxation and topiramate as controls. *Cephalalgia: An international journal of headache*, *31*(14), 1428–1438. https://doi.org/10.1177/0333102411419681

Vgontzas, A., & Pavlović, J. M. (2018). Sleep disorders and migraine: Review of literature and potential pathophysiology mechanisms. *Headache*, 58(7), 1030–1039. https://doi.org/10.1111/head.13358

United States Department of Health and Human Service. (2023). *Physical activity guidelines for Americans midcourse report: Implementation strategies for older adults.* https://health.gov/sites/default/files/2023-08/PAG_MidcourseReport_508c_08-10.pdf

Walker, W. H., Walton, J. C., DeVries, A. C., & Nelson, R. J. (2020). Circadian rhythm disruption and mental health. *Translational psychiatry*, *10*(1), 28. https://doi.org/10.1038/s41398-020-0694-0

Wang, Y., Wang, Y., Yue, G., Zhao, Y. (2023, April 13). Energy metabolism disturbance in migraine: From a mitochondrial point of view. *Frontiers in physiology*, 14. https://doi.org/10.3389/fphys.2023.1133528

Web MD Editorial Contributors (2022, January 26). *Silent migraines.* WebMD. https://www.webmd.com/migraines-headaches/what-are-silent-migraines

Wells, R. E., Burch, R., Paulsen, R. H., Wayne, P.M., Houle, T. T., &

Loder, E. (2014). Meditation for migraines: A pilot randomized controlled trial. *Headache: The journal of head and facepain*, 54: 1484-1495. https://doi.org/10.1111/head.12420

Westergaard, M. L., Hansen, E. H., Glümer, C., Olesen, J., & Jensen, R. H. (2014). Definitions of medication-overuse headache in population-based studies and their implications on prevalence estimates: a systematic review. *Cephalalgia: an international journal of headache*, *34*(6), 409–425. https://doi.org/10.1177/0333102413512033

What is migraine? (n.d.) National Migraine Centre. https://www.nationalmigrainecentre.org.uk/understanding-migraine/what-is-migraine/

Wong, S. H. (2024, April 4). Yoga for your brain? *Dr Sui Wong Empowering Your Brain Health Blog.* https://drsuiwongmd.blog/2024/04/04/yoga-for-your-brain/

The World Health Organization (WHO). (2011). *Global recommendation for physical activity on health.* https://www.who.int/docs/default-source/physical-activity/information-sheet-global-recommendations-on-physical-activity-for-health/physical-activity-recommendations-18-64years.pdf

Yablon LA, Mauskop A. *Magnesium in headache.* In: Vink R, Nechifor M, editors. Magnesium in the central nervous system. (2011). https://www.ncbi.nlm.nih.gov/books/NBK507271/

Zduńska, A., Cegielska, J., Zduński, S., & Domitrz, I. (2023). Caffeine for headaches: Helpful or harmful? A brief review of the literature. *Nutrients*, *15*(14), 3170. https://doi.org/10.3390/nu15143170

Printed in Great Britain
by Amazon

44314786R00099